Adolescent Medicine in the Middle East:
Principles, Perspectives, Practices

Asma J. Chattha • Samuel G. Porter
Philip R. Fischer

Adolescent Medicine in the Middle East: Principles, Perspectives, Practices

With Contributions from:
Nazleen Shakir Mala Ahmed
Alanoud Al-Ansari
Khadija Ali Alola
Yusur Turky Al Karaghouli
Vanitha A Jagannath
Madeeha Kamal
Huda Abu-Saad Huijer

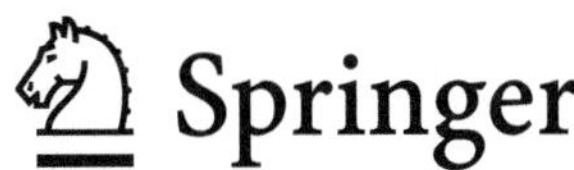 Springer

Asma J. Chattha
Department of Pediatric and Adolescent
Medicine
Mayo Clinic
Rochester, MN, USA

Samuel G. Porter
University of Kurdistan Hewler
Erbil, Iraq

Philip R. Fischer
International Advisory Services
Mayo Clinic
Rochester, MN, USA

ISBN 978-3-032-12347-3   ISBN 978-3-032-12348-0   (eBook)
https://doi.org/10.1007/978-3-032-12348-0

This Springer imprint is published by the registered company Springer Nature Switzerland AG
The registered company address is: Gewerbestrasse 11, 6330 Cham, Switzerland

If disposing of this product, please recycle the paper.

Introductions

Welcome to *Adolescent Medicine in the Middle East: Principles, Perspectives, and Practices*!

Together, we will use this book as a guide as we navigate a course toward helping adolescents prevent and overcome health problems. Our targeted outcome is healthy adults who have successfully completed their journeys through their adolescent years. We'll do this together, authors, commentators, and readers interacting along the way. This book can be a guide, a springboard, and a foundation for our mutual efforts to help teenagers gain and maintain good health.

Definitions

Many of us speak multiple languages, as do our patients. So, let's start with some definitions as we set a shared framework for this book.

"Adolescent Medicine" is the domain of health science that focuses on the prevention and treatment of diseases in individuals passing through the years between childhood and being adults. Typically, this involves dealing with individuals aged 10 to 20 years.

Originally, the term "Middle East" came from a British perspective as an empire expanded to increasingly more distant lands. The rest of Europe was considered "near" as colonizers and business dealers headed from their homeland; China and Southeast Asia were considered being "far" east of Britain. In-between was the vaguely delineated area called the "Middle East." Fortunately, we have advanced far beyond mere colonial and commercial interests, and we'll consider the Middle East to include the region from the shores of the eastern parts of the Mediterranean Sea (Turkey in the north, Egypt to the south, and the countries lining the eastern shores of the Mediterranean) through the lands of the Arabian Peninsula and Gulf Countries to the regions just west of India (including Afghanistan and Pakistan). Obviously, there are common similarities as well as vast differences among the people groups in this region, and this book should prove helpful in the care of *all* adolescents in this region.

Authors

Who are we, the main authors of this book?

Asma Chattha grew up and spent her adolescent years in Saudi Arabia, doing her medical studies at Aga Khan University in Pakistan. She is trained in pediatrics, pediatric endocrinology, and pediatric gynecology. She currently serves as an associate professor of pediatrics and the chair of reproductive health at Mayo Clinic Children's in the United States.

Sam Porter grew up and spent much of his adolescent years in Lebanon; he then went to medical school at the Mayo Clinic and did a family medicine residency in Wichita, Kansas, USA. He now works in Iraq.

Phil Fischer spent his adolescent and medical school years in California, USA. He has worked for 26 years with the Mayo Clinic, including being in the United Arab Emirates from 2020 to 2024 where he led adolescent medicine at Sheikh Shakhbout Medical City. He is a professor of pediatrics at Mayo Clinic and held a similar position at Khalifa University (in Abu Dhabi).

The authors of this book have collaboratively written medical articles and, individually, they account for hundreds of publications and hundreds of teaching sessions around the world. They share solid commitment to helping adolescents throughout the Middle East.

This Book

The purpose of this book is to facilitate excellent care of adolescents in the Middle East. It should be useful to medical students, resident physicians, pediatricians, internists, and family medicine physicians, as well as to nurses, psychologists, physical therapists, and dietitians. This book can be helpful to *anyone* involved in the care of adolescents.

This book is a result of teamwork, and the work of this team continues. The authors had helpful peer-review input from the collaborators. The collaborators added interesting sidebar comments. The publishing team made the book available. Now, you readers get to implement the care discussed in this book for the good of patients in the Middle East. Readers are invited to be participants, and correspondence is always welcome (to fischer.phil@mayo.edu).

As the subtitle (*Principles, Perspectives, and Practices*) suggests, this book is *not* intended to repeat all the medical information already available in other disease-based textbooks of pediatrics and family medicine. Rather, this book focuses on specific adolescent situations and issues while placing them into Middle Eastern contexts. This book provides an underlying approach to the care of all adolescents as well as tangible direction to guide the care of adolescents with common medical conditions.

Thanks for joining the process of improving adolescent health in the Middle East!

Contents

Chapter 1
Understanding and Communicating with Adolescents

Principles

Adolescence Is a Journey

Around ten years of age, a child is launched on to a journey. A child, dependent on others for daily life and just starting to develop a sense of personhood, is propelled forward. A decade later, an adult emerges, an adult with a unique personality and identity, an adult who can live independently, an adult ready to make important contributions to society.

The journey through the adolescent years can be wild and wonderful, dangerous and delightful, fun and frightful—all at the same time. A somewhat amorphous child is transformed into an adult with identity, independence, and importance.

Adolescence is an adventure. Adolescence is a journey to be shared. A growing child shares the delights and dangers of adolescence with individuals, families, and societies. Adolescence!

Concurrently, the adolescent is developing physically, emotionally, and psychosocially.

Physically, body composition is changing, especially related to size, muscle mass, and fat stores. Hormone levels are altered, sometimes with growing emotional variations. Emotionally, the emerging adolescent becomes ready for romance and, eventually, reproduction. Psychosocially, the boy or girl is developing identity, independence, and importance. Dealing with adolescents, we must understand and facilitate their journey, their process of becoming their future independent and valuable self.

Puberty! Puberty is the physical process by which a child's body becomes adult, with potential for sexual reproduction. For girls, breasts develop and enlarge. Pubic hair grows. Menses begin and become regular. Often slightly later than for girls, boys enter puberty, too. Their voices crack and deepen. Longitudinal growth

A. J. Chattha et al., *Adolescent Medicine in the Middle East: Principles, Perspectives, Practices*, https://doi.org/10.1007/978-3-032-12348-0_1

accelerates. Muscle mass expands. Hair shows up in new places. Genitals enlarge. For girls and for boys, skin changes, and acne can seem like a social disaster.

Puberty with its physical changes of adolescence simply happens. Children and their families can get excited or stressed, or they can simply observe passively. Their reactions to the bodily changes are important, but they can't do a lot to alter the normal processes.

Adolescence Is a Productive Process

As the adolescent's body is changing, the person growing through puberty is changing even more than is her or his body. Personalities deepen and expand as individual traits are established. Successful adolescent growth toward identity, independence, and importance is an interactive process; it requires favorable responses and input from the person, family, and society. We, as healthcare professionals, can significantly enhance a child's growth to adulthood, even if medical problems don't emerge along the way.

So, what are these processes? How does an *identity* get established? How is appropriate *independence* achieved? How can one develop *importance*? What is a clinician's role in all this? It is important that clinicians caring for adolescents understand answers to these questions.

Adolescents Are Discovering and Developing Identity

The beauty and the challenge of adolescence centers on *becoming*, on the development of a unique identity. Who will this person *become* and *be*? Will this individual be an athlete or a scholar or an artist? An introvert or an extrovert? How much of the identity will depend on gender, on race and ethnicity? How will this person relate to self, family, peers, authorities, and society? Adolescence is a journey of development and discovery of self, a process of gaining an understanding of the emerging self as it integrates in family and social networks.

Fostering Multi-faceted Identity Development

By nature, children are fairly self-centered. During adolescence, they discover their identities as unique individuals in relation to non-self, to family and to communities and to governmental structures and to God. The personal identity flourishes as it becomes integrated into people and purposes beyond the self.

Caring for adolescents, physicians have the privileges of recognizing what the patient is going through and of fostering success in the development of an individual identity, an individual identity that still incorporates relationships with others. We can ask questions and provide comments that might even help frame and guide the adolescent's development of identity.

Increasingly, some people believe that adolescents should choose their own identity, a bit like selecting food at a buffet. "You can be anything you want and do anything you want to do" is a refrain spread through personal conversations and graduation speeches. Clinicians can be cognizant of their personal moral values while remaining non-judgmental as they care for adolescents with evolving convictions. If a ten-year-old expresses fascination with death, enjoys killing insects and pets, and fantasizes about killing people, we would not encourage him or her to develop an identity as a murderer. If an adolescent who ambulates with difficulty due to cerebral palsy aspires to a career as a professional football player, we might encourage the interest in athletics while guiding a focus toward something more practically feasible. In some parts of the world, some clinicians believe that teens should be free to choose a gender and an identity as well as whether or not to be sexually promiscuous outside of a monogamous marriage. Clinicians, most of us would agree, can choose to have and to model principles that can help guide adolescents toward identities that contribute to their own health and to their healthy integration into society under the guidance of a transcendent Being. Clinicians need not impose their beliefs on adolescents, but they can model how they incorporate their own identities and beliefs into their daily lives.

Using Office Visits to Facilitate Tangible Development of Character, Convictions, and Identity

There are several aspects of this identity that is being developed during adolescence, and astute clinicians can incorporate identity development even into routine office visits. Our patients are developing concrete identities, with character and conviction; we can help them do so positively.

The adolescent identity is developing in specific, tangible, **concrete** ways, even with ongoing adjustments and flexibility. There are decisions to be made about academic focuses in school, athletic endeavors, and relationships. Clinicians can foster a growth mindset even while determining facts about relevant points of the social history. *What are your favorite subjects in school? How might you use that interest in a future job?* We can also help adolescents see daily life as a learning opportunity. *How was your summer vacation? As you traveled, what did you find was different about the culture there than what you are accustomed to here?* In our questioning, we get to know the adolescent and understand the context of her or his symptoms, but we also get to highlight the notions of growth and of developing and displaying a personal identity in concrete ways.

Adolescents are also developing **character**. Do they simply follow their peers, or do they think about the implications of their daily decisions? Will they hold to moral principles? Again, we can subtly encourage character development with simple questions. *What do most of your friends do with their free time? How does their focus on video games affect their success in school? How are you choosing to spend* *your time?* Quickly we learn about the patient, but we also demonstrate the value of thoughtfully making decisions that will lead to wise character development. *Yes, lots of teenagers think their siblings are annoying. How do you choose to respond when you are bugged by your sister?* Simple questions help teens see that even in an imperfect world they have the option to behave responsibly.

Adolescents are also developing **convictions**, beliefs that will frame their lives. Self-centered as teens, they are growing to increasingly focus on the needs of others. *What was going on in your peer's life to make him spread bad rumors about you? How have your parents modeled dealing with adversity? What do you learn in your faith community about dealing with evil in the world?* We don't need long responses or long discussions, but our simple questions point our patients to see their daily lives in the context of their emerging identities—becoming their concrete selves with solid character and sensible convictions. Obviously, all this ties in directly to them choosing healthy habits about diet and exercise, substance use, and peer relationships that will help prepare them for a healthy entry into adult life.

> **Conversation and Reflection**
> Questions about role models, challenges, and values during routine adolescent visits can spark meaningful conversations. They help youth reflect on who they want to become, beyond academics or sports.
>
> Nazleen Shakir Mala Ahmed, MBChB, MS, FKBMS
> Erbil, Iraq

Identity Development Through Experimentation

Sometimes adolescents "test the waters" in asserting a personal identity by trying activities that are the opposite of what parents and authorities might suggest. They might seek to join in with peers with whom they share or aspire to share specific interests and identities. Trying to fit in to their new emerging selves, they might actually alienate themselves from other people and make themselves even less comfortable with their own emerging identities. Experimentation, whether with illicit substances or improper relationships, might lead to persistent bad habits; this identity formation might have negative consequences. Parents and clinicians should be comfortable going through some of these adolescent challenges, expressing love and compassion for the individual but not encouraging or condoning improper activities. Again, asking reflective questions can help the teen learn to keep a "search for self" in line with acceptable societal restrictions on some behaviors.

Non-traditional Identities

It's important to recognize that not all adolescents fit traditional gender, cultural, or family molds. As family physicians, we can create a safe space for teens to express who they are without fear of judgment.

Nazleen Shakir Mala Ahmed, MBChB, MS, FKBMS
Erbil, Iraq

Adolescents Are Developing Independence

Young children depend on adults. Young children need other people to provide them with food, beverage, and safety. They need people to give them places to sleep and to play and to learn. Young children are dependent.

Adults are independent members of an inter-connected society. They have been educated and experienced in ways that make it possible for them to provide much of their own sustenance and safe accommodations. They can gain employment, generate income, and contribute to the needs of society.

Adolescents are no longer totally dependent children, and yet they are not yet independent adults. A key feature of the adolescent years is the process of developing independence.

Like identity, independence is housed within the contexts of family, peers, communities, and God. In addition, adolescents' opportunities to build independence can differ dramatically depending on social class, gender roles, and cultural norms. All independence is within a broader context of ongoing dependence on groups of people and a transcendent Being.

So, how does an emerging adolescent begin to develop independence?

Adolescents want to make their own decisions, but they also want to fit in with their peer group. As they take initial steps of independence from their parents, they are still dependent on the affirmation and advice of their peers. Whether related to hair style, clothing choices, or activity preferences, adolescents test their independence by making choices of which their parents might not approve. At the same time, their choices are often planned to give them credibility and connection with their peers. Wise parents (and wise clinicians) can help adolescents make informed choices as they exercise their growing independence.

Adolescents also explore their own interests, interests that might not align with parental preferences. They might choose newer styles of music. They might target career options that vary from what their parents did. The choice of friends and peer groups offers another opportunity to express independence. Again, parents and clinicians can recognize the value of these moves toward independence, and they can foster good choices along the way.

Evolving independence rightly comes with limits. Adolescents might want more complete control than that for which they are actually prepared. Good parents can help ensure that adolescents heading out, to a mall with peers perhaps, do so with enough funds to meet needs and reasonable desires but not with excessive funds that might lead to inappropriate independent spending. Emerging adolescents can learn to accept limits to independence, and they will someday appreciate that adults helped them decide which drivers were adequately safe to be entrusted with transporting the adolescent.

Conflict is normal as adolescents struggle to balance their emerging independence with wise and safe decision-making. Appropriate independence is not just self-sufficiency; rather, appropriate independence is a capacity to support and manage one's self while living in the context of a family and society that help ensure the good of a population.

Choices of friends and peer groups, like learning good safety and healthy behaviors, offer adolescents with good opportunity both to succeed and to fail as they learn appropriate independence.

Thinking About Peer Influences

Peers have a strong influence on adolescents' independence-related decisions, from hairstyles to risky behaviors. Encouraging teens to reflect on their choices helps build self-awareness and confidence.

Nazleen Shakir Mala Ahmed, MBChB, MS, FKBMS
Erbil, Iraq

Adolescents Are Sensing Importance, or at Least They Want To

Adolescence is, in part, a process of moving from self-centeredness to others-orientation. The early teen sometimes struggles between feeling like the center of the world, on one hand, and an inconsequential nothing, on the other. Adolescents grow toward an appropriate understanding of importance.

Important or Invisible

In my practice, adolescents often fluctuate between thinking they are the center of the world and feeling invisible. Supporting their growth toward balanced self-worth, including valuing their contributions to others, can help build resilience.

Nazleen Shakir Mala Ahmed, MBChB, MS, FKBMS
Erbil, Iraq

Importance refers to a positive sense of self that is appropriately related to others. The adolescent is valuable and should, appropriately sense personal value, worth, and esteem. At the same time, this internal sense of importance empowers the adolescent to contribute positively to the lives of others. The adolescent develops abilities to contribute to society in ways that are important to the community.

We believe that the adolescent should develop appropriate senses of self-esteem and self-efficacy.

Initially, adolescents might think that everyone else is or should be as concerned about them as they are themselves. They might think that others are seeing the tiny forehead pimple as a near-volcanic eruption. Or, they might think that others will assume a bad grade on an exam indicates that the person is bad. As the teenage years progress, adolescents come to see themselves as having importance and dignity as individuals but also as having importance through their relationships with others. Then, they seek to align themselves with "greater goods," with activities and aspirations that produce benefit for other people.

When discussing options with adolescents, whether about a career or about how to spend an evening, supportive adults can help the adolescent grow from a perspective of "what will I get out of this" to concern for "how can I be useful to others." The teen needs to grow to see value and importance in self and then to use that to engage with others in important ways.

Appropriate Praise
Praising a teen's effort and character, rather than only their achievements, encourages a growth mindset. This is key to fostering confidence and motivation.

Nazleen Shakir Mala Ahmed, MBChB, MS, FKBMS
Erbil, Iraq

Thought processes will mature in a growing adolescent as she or he senses importance not just in doing but in being. Adults can increasingly commend teens for the importance of the person they are becoming. For instance, it might not be adequate to focus on the accomplishment by saying something like "you scored better on the exam this time than last time;" it might be better to comment on the person behind the accomplishment, on the being beyond the doing, with a comment like "your performance on that exam demonstrates that you are the sort of person that has commitment and a willingness to work diligently." We can help growing adolescents sense appropriate importance for who they are and for who they are becoming. It is often more effective in the long run to commend teens for their underlying attitude than simply for their overt actions.

Then, adolescents grow to sense importance beyond their individual selves by seeing importance by their associations with a larger "whole." They learn to link their personal value and importance to the value of their community and their purposes and their God. Their sense of importance expands even as their sense of perspective expands—from self to family to community to God.

> **Limited Autonomy**
> In my family practice in the Middle East, many adolescents still rely heavily on their parents for healthcare decisions. Acknowledging this dependence while still giving teens a voice helps foster gradual, culturally respectful autonomy.
>
> Nazleen Shakir Mala Ahmed, MBChB, MS, FKBMS
> Erbil, Iraq

Perspectives from the Middle East

Of course, generalizations are dangerous! In various settings in the Middle East, as elsewhere in the world, even the definition of "adolescence" varies. Some pediatricians care only for children up to age 12 years, and others have been trained to care for patients into their early 20s. Sadly, though, some adolescents in certain settings feel like they don't fit; they don't sense a welcome into either a pediatric or an adult medical practice. In recent years, though, many medical settings in the Gulf states and other Middle Eastern settings have expanded the definition of "pediatrics" to include the care of children up to at least 16 or 18 years of age. Of course, generalists and family physicians seeing patients of all ages can readily welcome adolescents into their practices.

The field of Adolescent Medicine is much different in some Middle Eastern settings than it is in North America and Europe. In the Middle East, "adolescent medicine" frequently deals with the management of chronic illness and the enhancement of reproductive health. In Europe and North America, the field of Adolescent Medicine has developed a strong focus on issues related to sexuality, substance use, and mood disorders.

Clearly, many North Americans grew up with a strong sense of individuality. Nations began with rebellion against authority, and individuals rose by their own effort. In some Middle Eastern settings, there is a much greater sense of community behind the development of identity, independence, and importance. One of the pleasures of working with adolescents is that of seeing wholesome inter-personal and in-group relationships developing as adolescents gain culturally appropriate senses of who they are and how they fit into the world. Community in some Middle Eastern settings implies that even adolescents and married young adults are not independent from the daily demands of their parents or parents-in-law.

There are regional and sub-cultural variations in the appropriateness of physical touch in the Middle East. In general, greeting pediatric patients with a high-five or a fist bump can provide an effective and fun personal connection. By the middle adolescent years, however, some females reject such a physical greeting (and even more so a handshake) from a male physician. Shaking hands of a different gender parent would also feel invasive and inappropriate. Similarly, placing an empathetic hand on the shoulder of a patient or parent would not be favorably accepted, even though that gesture would be welcomed and appreciated by non-Muslim patients and parents in some other parts of the world. Greetings involving touch should be considered carefully and individually since preferences vary throughout the region.

What should clinicians new to the Middle East do? Relevant guidance for dealing with adolescents in many Middle Eastern settings includes clear guidance: (1) ask before you touch, (2) involve parents appropriately, and, (3) when communicating with adolescents and their families, be cognizant of cultural aspects of gender dynamics.

Practices in the Middle East

Communicating with Adolescents

So what? Does this understanding of adolescent development impact our interactions with adolescents and their families? Yes, totally!

Thus, based on a proper understanding of adolescence, there are concrete recommendations about how to communicate with adolescents. There are clear implications that affect every detail of each medical encounter.

Initial Contact

Greetings

Adolescents are very discerning. Within a few nanoseconds of meeting someone, adolescents have often decided if they like and trust the person they are meeting. Since most treatments of adolescents require behavioral change (whether taking medication or getting exercise or adjusting a diet) and since behavior change is more likely when the adolescent likes and trusts the clinician providing treatment, it is essential that we do what we can to bond well, to develop a good therapeutic alliance.

The quality of the therapeutic alliance we build depends in good measure on how well adolescents sense that we value their identity, that we provide them independence, and that we consider them important.

Entering a room where the patient is waiting? Knock and enter slowly, gently. Rushing in suggests that you don't really value the person enough to give unhurried time.

Is the patient coming in to a room where you are? Rise to greet the person, demonstrating that you value and respect their importance.

> **The Initial Moments Together**
> In my clinic, I've found that how you begin the first 30 s with an adolescent sets the tone for the entire encounter. A warm smile and a patient-centered opening often lead to better disclosure, especially around sensitive topics.
>
> Nazleen Shakir Mala Ahmed, MBChB, MS, FKBMS
> Erbil, Iraq

Introductions

Make eye contact, with the adolescent before you look at the parent. This shows that you prioritize the person and grant the adolescent a sense of independence even as you, secondarily, will demonstrate interest in and respect for the parent, too. Be genuinely welcoming.

> **Details Matter**
> Even small gestures—like avoiding physical barriers or making eye contact before turning to the parent—send a strong signal that the teen is being seen and heard as an individual.
>
> Nazleen Shakir Mala Ahmed, MBChB, MS, FKBMS
> Erbil, Iraq

Many young physicians are taught to first introduce themselves. There is good reason for that, but your attire and nametag and setting will likely give the patient a clue about who you are. And, if you start by talking about yourself, the patient will quickly jump to the conclusion that this encounter is more about you than about the patient. It's better to confirm the patient's identity first, showing that the patient is the priority in the room. If you know, for instance, that you are seeing a 15-year-old girl for chronic abdominal pain, your initial words will be about the patient rather than about yourself. Perhaps you can even ask if this person is the resilient 15-year-old you've heard about; if she looks puzzled, you can explain that you understand she has been tolerating terrible discomfort for a long time and still pursuing recovery. In so doing, you have identified her as the patient, you have validated the legitimacy of her symptoms, you have commended her for being as tolerant and strong as she is, and you have already pointed the outcome of the encounter toward recovery.

Then, after those few seconds to identify the patient, you can say that you are so happy that you get to be part of the team caring for her. Your value is found in helping the patient, and the patient, by now, feels important and central to the interaction. You have not bored (and lost) the patient with a lengthy description of your name and title and role, but you have affirmed the patient and stated your desire to find value in being of help.

Roles and Relationships

Having established the importance of the patient as an independent individual, you can then ask who the other person in the room is. Especially in collective cultures such as in the Middle East, it is crucial to acknowledge the adolescent's voice while still engaging the parent as a supportive partner in care. Even in the initial 20 seconds of the interaction, we have provided affirmation of the identity (resilient), independence (primary communicator), and importance (worthy of support and help from you and from the parent) of the patient. At the same time, we have validated the parent as important to us and to the patient. If you've done all this with a warmly welcoming, genuine smile in an unhurried fashion, you have already succeeded in establishing a good therapeutic alliance!

Organize the Physical Environment

Through this beginning of the encounter, you will pay attention to other important details. It is usually helpful to avoid demonstrations of power that will alienate the patient—ensure eye contact at eye level, avoid tables or desks separating you from the patient, and act relaxed. Keep yourself close enough to the patient to show interest but not so close as to invade his or her comfort zone. Keep the parent within eyesight, but maintain direct connection to the patient. Make adjustments as you see the patient withdraw or cross arms or get nervous.

Getting the History

From the outset, we should clarify what goals the patient has for the medical encounter. Our explanations will be different if the main goal is to "know what is going on" than if the goal is "to stop hurting." We need to identify the patient's (and family's) goals in order to customize our explanation of the evaluation and treatment plan.

Context is important. While getting the specific details of the key symptoms and the course of the present illness, we also need to fit the symptoms into the context of the patient's life. This helps us understand the severity and consequences of the symptoms and allows us to understand the life situation into which treatment will be added. One way to cover the context is to use a memory aid such as HEADS to remind us to learn about **H**ome situation, **E**ducational setting, **A**ctivities with which the patient is engaged, **D**rugs and medications the patient uses, **S**ocial situations including sexual activity, support structures, and suicidal thoughts or other signs of depression or anxiety. (There is more detailed discussion of the HEADS assessment tool in Chap. 2 on Routine Care of Adolescents.) Otherwise stated, we want to understand the *identity* of the patient—what the patient does and what the patient cares about, how the patient sees himself or herself fitting into friend groups and society, and what the patient wants to do in the future.

Sometimes, we need to talk with the patient separately from the parent. This is routine and normal, so we don't really want to ask for permission as if it is unusual. Rather, we might ask the parent "Is there anything else you'd like me to know before I talk with your child alone?" While parents in some Middle Eastern settings hesitate to leave an adolescent alone with a clinician, many will agree when they realize this is routine in the standard care of an adolescent. If the patient and I are of different genders, I would include a chaperone (perhaps a nurse) of the same gender as the patient to talk about issues that might initially seem uncomfortable.

Even when we have bonded well with the patient and think we have developed the beginnings of a good therapeutic alliance, the patient might hesitate to disclose personal facts about sexuality and substance use. Rather than ask directly what the patient does, I initially express my ignorance about the patient's school situation and ask how common it is for classmates to engage in whatever activity I want to discuss. If the patient seems embarrassed and says "hardly anyone," it is unlikely that the patient is involved with that activity. But, if the patient casually responds that "most of my classmates are doing it," I would assume that at least this patient's close peer group is involved and that the patient probably is, too. I can then gently lead into "and what about you" while asking what the patient does in that area, making it clear that I won't tell the parents unless I think someone's life is at risk.

> **Opening Personal Communication**
> Adolescents are more likely to open up when questions are phrased indirectly, such as asking what's common in their school or among peers. This lowers defensiveness and helps build trust.
>
> Nazleen Shakir Mala Ahmed, MBChB, MS, FKBMS
> Erbil, Iraq

Especially when talking about substance use and sexuality, we want to openly welcome whatever the patient has to say to us. We don't want to be harsh and judgmental. At the same time, we can make it clear that we have our own personal ideas about what is right but that we value the patient and will care for him or her no matter what the patient is doing. On one hand, we don't want to close the conversation with wording like "you don't ever do this do you" but we also don't want to encourage behavior by saying "how often do you do this" in a way that will leave the patient feeling abnormal for not engaging in the behavior we are discussing. I heard of one girl who thought maybe she *should* be having sex since three doctors in a row had asked how many partners she had.

There are rules about confidentiality and privacy in some settings that legislate how a physician should communicate with an adolescent about sensitive issues. There are also conservative cultural traditions in some areas that limit open disclosure but also limit keeping information from families. Within the limits of the setting, though, the physician will at least let the patient know that their conversation is "safe" and that details will only be revealed to others if truly necessary. Wisely, some clinicians prefer to explicitly discuss issues of confidentiality with the patient and family together before entering into discussion of sensitive topics.

Doing the Exam

If the same-gender parent is not in the room with us, we should have a chaperone of the same gender as the patient in the room when we are talking about potentially uncomfortable topics and when we are doing an undressed physical exam. Some parts of the history are comfortably done while concurrently doing the physical exam. Of course, the patient should never feel uncomfortably exposed, and we should maintain modesty.

In some cultural settings, staff and sometimes other patients open doors to enter exam rooms while an exam is in progress. Validating the importance of the patient, we should be willing to lock doors and avoid interruptions. Curtains should keep the patient out of view of family members (and windows!) during an exam. Gowns or sheets should keep body parts covered when they are not being examined. And, respecting patients, we should provide for same gender examiners when requested. We validate patients when we maintain their privacy. At the same time, in some Middle Eastern settings, exams of the body surface are not common, and some clinics don't even keep gowns available. While respecting the patient's modesty and privacy, we should still ensure that an adequate physical exam is completed.

Explaining the Plan

When talking about diagnoses, testing, and treatment, keep centered on the patient's goal(s). Explain what the patient wanted to know and how the tests and/or treatment help meet the patient's goal(s), even if you expand the explanation to go beyond the initial basic goals of the patient.

Circle Back
When discussing treatment, always circle back to the teen's original concern. Linking our plan to their personal goals helps build motivation and follow-through.

Nazleen Shakir Mala Ahmed, MBChB, MS, FKBMS
Erbil, Iraq

Therapeutic Alliance

By showing respect for the patient during the initial minutes of each encounter, we are able to better engage the patient in the process of the evaluation, and we are more likely to find that patients trust our input and comply with our treatment recommendations. Developing a therapeutic alliance requires concerted attention, but it doesn't require much additional time; and good patient engagement fosters recovery.

For Reflection
A 2020 article by Sunde and colleagues in *Pediatrics in Review* (cited below) proposed 16 features organized under five themes of good interaction with adolescents who have chronic symptoms (connection, collaboration, comprehension, coordination, and communication), along with illustrative examples. These same ideas are relevant for any clinical encounter with a symptomatic adolescent. Consider how to incorporate specific words and actions into your next patient encounter to facilitate successful interactions.

Further Reading

1. Sunde KE, Hilliker DR, Fischer PR. Understanding and managing adolescents with conversion and functional disorders. Pediatr Rev. 2020;41(12):630–41. https://doi.org/10.1542/pir.2019-0042.
2. Moreno M, Thompson L. What is adolescent and young adult medicine? JAMA Pediatr. 2020 May 1;174(5):512. https://doi.org/10.1001/jamapediatrics.2020.0311.

Chapter 2
Routine Care of Adolescents

Principles

Routine visits can help a clinician give input into lifestyle and career choices adolescents are facing.

We have already said that a key feature of adolescence is the development of identity, independence, and importance. During episodic health maintenance visits, a good clinician can be updated about the developing adolescent's interests and progress toward adulthood. With an ongoing relationship, the adolescent can hear input from a caring clinician about lifestyle and career choices. Routine visits offer opportunities to guide healthy adolescent development.

A clinician who stays in contact with an adolescent is more likely to be trusted with personal information when concerns arise.

As adolescents move toward independence, they can become at least temporarily skeptical about the role of adults in their lives. Trust is unlikely to come just because of the clinician's professional role. Rather, having a history of showing interest in the adolescent, the clinician finds the adolescent to be more open to share thoughts about personal issues and, then, to be more open to the clinician's input.

Standardized screening can identify emerging issues when early intervention can be effective.

Not all pending health concerns are obvious to the adolescent, the adolescent's family, or to a clinician during a brief visit. Standardized screening tools allow clinicians to identify areas of potential concern. Even adolescents who "seem normal" might not be doing as well as they superficially appear to be. Adolescents unwilling to abruptly raise mental health issues will still likely be willing to accurately respond to standardized screening questions about anxiety and depression. Routinely posing standardized questions about health, education, activities, depression, and

A. J. Chattha et al., *Adolescent Medicine in the Middle East: Principles, Perspectives, Practices*, https://doi.org/10.1007/978-3-032-12348-0_2

socialization (such as by using the HEADS assessment, discussed below) can allow for ongoing conversation about important issues. Standardized gathering of important data can facilitate identification of pending concerns while facilitating good lifestyle choices.

Addressing Body Image and Eating Practices
Body dissatisfaction and unhealthy weight control practices are increasingly common among adolescents in the Middle East. Routine care or illness visits can serve as valuable opportunities for early detection. Using brief screening tools, such as the SCOFF questionnaire,* allows for early identification and timely referral for support.

Alanoud Al-Ansari, MD, MHPE
Doha, Qatar

* https://pmc.ncbi.nlm.nih.gov/articles/PMC1070794/

Regular physical exams provide opportunity for adolescents to discuss their own physical development and growth.

Similarly, standardized assessment of physical findings is important to identify pending physical problems that might not yet be clinically evident. At least annually, adolescents should have height and weight measured (with calculation of body mass index) as well as blood pressure. Abnormal findings can prompt further evaluation. A hands-on physical exam can identify other important findings that the adolescent might not have recognized—acanthosis nigricans with concern for problems of glucose metabolism, thyromegaly with concern for hypothyroidism, scoliosis that would be helped by early diagnosis and intervention, and Tanner staging done respectfully to identify concerns about hormonal development. At the same time, talking about normal findings on a physical exam might help reassure patients, such as an adolescent boy with benign physiologic gynecomastia, even if the patient had not been willing to voice a concern about that finding. Conversation during the course of the physical exam can use positive and negative findings as the basis for discussion of concerns and of healthy behavioral choices.

Seeing patients repeatedly during the adolescent years provides clinicians with the opportunity to impact the development of good lifestyle choices.

Adolescents are incorporating lifestyle choices into daily living. Following growth and activities (such as with the HEADS assessment) provides opportunity for interactive discussion that commends the adolescent for healthy choices about diet, sleep, and exercise. Asking about the duration of daily non-educational screen time opens the door toward discussion about motivations behind "social" activities and how the adolescent can be empowered to make wise choices. In regions where substance abuse and sexual activity are common during adolescence, regular health maintenance visits make discussion of these topics routine, in a socially acceptable and respectful fashion.

Staying current on recommended vaccinations is one of the most effective ways to prevent serious health problems.

Vaccines save lives. Even after the initial childhood series of routine vaccines, additional vaccinations can help prevent common diseases. Routine check-up visits provide a good opportunity to ensure that routine vaccination is up-to-date.

Good communication is critically important.

Cultural conservatism makes some conversations challenging for adolescents, especially when the patient and clinician are of different genders. In the course of conversation about the HEADS assessment topics, however, it is socially appropriate and easy for a clinician to ask the adolescent about common social practices at the patient's school. For instance, instead of starting a discussion about substance abuse (or any other sensitive topic) with blunt questions such as "do you use illegal drugs," the clinician might ask curiosity questions such as "in your school, how common is it for your classmates to smoke." That question about other people in general is not personally threatening and is easier, for the adolescent, to answer conversationally. Other detailed questions can follow, and then the clinician can get more personally relevant with "What about your closest friends? Are some of them smoking?" Then, the clinician can ask for the adolescent's view of such behaviors. Confidentiality is key, and adolescents find it easier to provide honest information when questions do not seem personally threatening.

Perspectives from the Middle East

There is a huge variation in the availability of health care maintenance visits for adolescents in the Middle East. In some areas, there are no regularly scheduled check-ups for adolescents. In other areas, annual visits are routine for healthy adolescents. In some settings, only athletes receive pre-participation check-ups. Sometimes, the availability of adolescent check-ups varies with the payment possibilities for patients; when adolescent health care maintenance visits are not routine for individuals with government insurance funding, they are available for individuals able to pay for this optional sort of care. Increasingly, there is an emphasis on "longevity clinics," and adolescent check-ups are completely consistent with that sort of care, with or without testing for genetic risk factors.

Especially in areas where obesity is common, as well as in areas where substance abuse is growing, there is increased interest in having adolescents seen regularly. As science advances, especially following the COVID-19 pandemic, there is broad interest in maintaining and enhancing health, even in those who seem to be well.

In some areas where visits for healthy-seeming adolescents are not routine, clinicians have found it useful to do screening at the time of visits for illness. Identification of abnormal growth trajectories or mental health concerns or under-immunization can then prompt subsequent appointments to deal specifically with the identified concerns.

> **Including Refugee Adolescents in Health Maintenance**
> Adolescents displaced by conflict are a vulnerable group across the Middle East. Although many are integrated into local schools and do not face language barriers, access to routine healthcare may be limited by financial constraints or lack of awareness. Mental health screening is especially important, as these adolescents may carry unaddressed trauma and emotional distress.
>
> Alanoud Al-Ansari, MD, MHPE
> Doha, Qatar

With some subpopulations of adolescents in the Middle East, any discussion related to male-female relationships is best handled carefully by a clinician of the same sex as the patient. Similarly, some clinicians choose to leave even discrete Tanner staging for same-sex clinicians. While modesty is important, a healthcare team should not allow concerns for privacy to allow important discussions and exam findings to be missed.

Similarly, confidentiality is nuanced in the Middle East as compared to the situation in other countries. Parents often want to be present for all clinician interactions with older adolescents. Honesty with patients and family members is important, but adolescents with concerns about mental health or sexuality or substance use might be more willing to discuss these issues without parental presence. Parents are usually willing to allow private clinician-patient discussions once they know that the clinician, with the parent, is working toward the patient becoming an independent adult and once the parent is assured that life-endangering health problems would have to be disclosed to the parent.

While some topics might be considered taboo by some patients and parents, careful explanation by a compassionate and confident clinician can usually help families agree to the value of confidential care for adolescents. The risk of avoiding taboo topics is that the patient might not receive necessary care that could prevent undesired consequences of the adolescent's "taboo" behavior.

Practices in the Middle East

Make a plan to ensure that every adolescent receives appropriate health maintenance interventions, whatever the setting.

Not every practice setting will be conducive to offering routine health care maintenance visits for adolescents. But, every clinician can at least incorporate key aspects
of health promotion, disease prevention, and injury prevention into regular visits for
illness.

Height and weight should be measured at least every six months during the adolescent years, and this can quickly be done during acute care visits; any identified
growth concerns can prompt the scheduling of a follow-up visit for that concern.
Even a quick exam during an illness-related visit can make note of significant pallor,
acanthosis, thyromegaly, or an abdominal mass. While placing the stethoscope on
the skin of the anterior chest or the hands on the lower abdomen for palpitation, it is
possible to at least approximate a Tanner score. Quick questions can provide updates
about school, sport, and social activities.

The vaccine record can be scanned, and plans can be made to provide any necessary vaccinations. Of course, this implies that the clinician has set up an adequate
record system so growth curves and immunization records are readily available.

National immunization schedules vary depending on the local epidemiology of
vaccine-preventable diseases and on the feasibility of providing vaccines. With
many adolescents and young adults traveling, it might also be important to provide
vaccines against additional illnesses that are not present in the home region. General
guidance about vaccines that could be relevant for adolescents follow, and current
detailed recommendations from the World Health Organization, Centers for Disease
Control and Prevention, and national health authorities can be consulted online:

1. Routine Childhood Vaccines. Obviously, what is "routine" varies from place to
   place. But, every adolescent should be protected against diphtheria, tetanus, and
   pertussis. Since pertussis immunity wanes within a decade after the most recent
   vaccine, many adolescents are due for a booster dose of diphtheria, tetanus, and
   pertussis vaccination.
2. Polio. The childhood series of polio vaccine should be completed during adolescence if it was not completed earlier.
3. Hepatitis B. The initial series of three hepatitis B vaccines should be completed
   during adolescence if it was not completed earlier.
4. Varicella. If the adolescent has managed not to develop varicella and was not
   immunized, it would be wise to provide varicella vaccination during adolescence. This is especially true since complications of varicella are more common
   in adults than in younger children.
5. Measles, mumps, and rubella. Measles is, again, increasingly common in many
   areas of the world. A single vaccine prior to one year of age protects about 60%
   of recipients against measles, yet many others are left unprotected. Appropriate
   protection comes with two separate measles-mumps-rubella vaccines at least a
   month apart after 12 months of age. Girls who have not had rubella illness or
   vaccine should receive the measles-mumps-rubella vaccine before contemplat-
   ing pregnancy, so an adolescent vaccine can be very appropriate.

6. Pneumococcus. The childhood series of pneumococcal vaccine should be provided to all children. Adolescents with chronic pulmonary or immunologic disorders might benefit from additional pneumococcal vaccines.
7. Influenza. Annual influenza vaccine can prevent illness during adolescence. Patients with asthma and other chronic lung conditions can be especially helped by this vaccine.
8. COVID-19. Even after the pandemic, adolescents should receive vaccinations as indicated by health authorities.
9. Hepatitis A. Hepatitis A is more severe in older children and adults than in younger children. With improving sanitation and hygiene, hepatitis A has become less common during childhood. A single vaccine dose given after one year of age protects almost all recipients for at least ten years. Thus, it is sensible that all adolescents who have not previously received hepatitis A vaccination receive a single dose of hepatitis A vaccine.
10. Human Papillomavirus. Human papilloma virus infection leads to cancer, especially in females, and asymptomatic males can transmit the infection to intimate partners. Unless it can be guaranteed that an individual will never have sexual contact with a non-virgin, this vaccine should be provided at least to all girls during early adolescence. Depending on age and the specific vaccine used, a two or three dose series is effective.
11. Meningococcus. Meningitis and sepsis due to meningococcus B are more common in North America and Europe. Illness due to meningococcus A (as well as C, Y, and W) are more common in the Middle East, Africa, and Asia. Vaccination is effective but is usually given only to those with specific geographic risks (such as going on a pilgrimage to Mecca or moving to North America for university studies).
12. Dengue. Some adolescents moving to dengue-endemic regions should be vaccinated. Current health authority guidelines should be consulted since these vaccines are relatively new and their use depends on the individual's previous exposure to dengue virus.
13. Typhoid. This vaccine can be useful for adolescents traveling to or through some resource-limited areas. An intramuscular dose protects for two years; the oral vaccine series protects for five years.
14. Yellow Fever. This vaccine is important prior to travel to some areas of South America and Africa. A single dose given at or after nine months of age provides life-long protection.
15. Japanese Encephalitis Virus. This vaccine is useful for people who will be spending more than a month in rural areas that are endemic for this infection, especially in areas with pig farming.

At least annually, even during an illness visit, screening for anxiety and depression can be done. Simple, validated questionnaires are available online, as discussed in Chap. 6. The PHQ-9 questionnaire for depression and the GAD-7 questionnaire for anxiety can be completed in the waiting room if the patient is not excessively compromised by the acute illness that prompted the visit. However, it behooves the clinician to review the results before the patient leaves the visit and, if needed for elevated/abnormal results, to promptly arrange appropriate follow-up care.

Confidentiality in Adolescent Care
Adolescents are more likely to share sensitive concerns when they trust that their privacy is respected. Explaining the purpose and limits of confidentiality helps build that trust with both adolescents and their parents. In my experience, most parents in the Middle East (even if initially hesitant) accept brief private conversations when asked gently and respectfully, especially when framed as supporting the adolescent's independence.

Alanoud Al-Ansari, MD, MHPE
Doha, Qatar

The HEADS assessment provides a framework to learn about a patient beyond the degree of a typical past history and review of systems. There are various online versions of the HEADS (or HEADSS) assessment, and the details of the categories and the exact questions are not nearly as important as that the major points are discussed. However, many clinicians find it helpful to keep a simple mnemonic in mind to facilitate completeness of discussion with adolescents. The questions can be asked in a formal structured manner, but many clinicians prefer to gather the information with a more conversational style. By whatever fashion, at least each year a clinician should be updated by an adolescent about the **h**ome situation, where the adolescent is and where he or she plans to go **e**ducationally and with **e**mployment, what **a**ctivities (social, sports, hobbies, extra-curricular organizations) are important to the patient, whether there are concerns for **d**epression (the patient's view, in addition to the PHQ-9), whether **d**rugs/substances are being used or considered (including nutritional supplements and over-the-counter products as well as smoking and vaping which are increasingly common in some Middle East settings), what male-female relationships are part of the patient's life (and, if relevant, concerns about gender identity and **s**exual activity), **s**afety precautions (use of seat belts in four-wheeled vehicles and use of helmets when on a bicycle, motorcycle, or scooter), and ways the adolescent chooses to manage **s**ocial media activity. Clinicians will want to customize their approach with adolescents as they cover relevant topics, and the HEADS mnemonic might help—even though not all bold-print letters in this description (HEEADDSSSS) need be used as separate categories. Many clinicians simply try to remember to discuss **h**ome, **e**ducation, **a**ctivities, **d**rugs, and **s**ocial situations. Information gathered is useful to: (1) maintain a good physician-patient relationship that is useful to encourage and guide ongoing development of identity, independence, and importance, and, (2) identify topics that raise concern for active risk that should be pursued in more detail.

Asking About the Use of Contraceptive Pills
In many Middle Eastern countries, contraceptive pills (often called hormonal pills by adolescents) are available over the counter. In my practice, adolescents often don't mention them when asked about medications, but do when specifically asked about non-prescription use. Including this in routine screening can create space for nonjudgmental conversations about relationships and sexuality.

Alanoud Al-Ansari, MD, MHPE
Doha, Qatar

See every adolescent visit as an opportunity to help develop identity, independence, and importance.

Even greetings and introductory small-talk comments can be part of helpful information gathering *and* encouragement of the patient's ongoing development from childhood through adolescence to adulthood. Documenting the patient's key interests in the medical record can prompt personalized conversation at subsequent visits.

Open a door to discuss any patient concerns about pubertal changes.

Pubertal changes of hair growth, genital size, voice quality, and acne can be frightening to patients. It helps if clinicians raise puberty as a normal part of life and use open-ended questions to help the adolescent express even private concerns. "You're 13 now," the clinician might say, "and into puberty. How's that going? What of all the body changes is most fun, and what is most concerning?"

Provide care coordination and appropriate transitions.

Caring for adolescents is not a solo endeavor. Clinicians should consciously engage with families, school personnel, and other clinicians as appropriate for each patient.

Adolescents with chronic or complex problems can benefit from a coordinating clinician that can guide subspecialty input and treatment. This coordinating clinician plays a key role in interpreting, synthesizing, and applying subspecialty input in ways that are most helpful to the patient and family.

Adolescents eventually become adults. Especially for those with chronic conditions who will only achieve limited independence, it is important for the adolescent clinician to ensure an effective transition to adult-focused clinicians and services. Warm hand-offs by which the patient, family, adolescent clinician, and adult specialists meet together can facilitate effective transitions for particularly complex patients.

For Reflection
In your current setting, what practical changes can be made to ensure that adolescents best receive good health promotion and preventive care?

Further Reading

1. World Health Organization. Routine Immunizations. https://www.who.int/teams/immunization-vaccines-and-biologicals/policies/who-recommendations-for-routine-immunization%2D%2D-summary-tables
2. Centers for Disease Control and Prevention. Child and Adolescent Immunization Schedule by Age. https://www.cdc.gov/vaccines/hcp/imz-schedules/child-adolescent-age.html

Chapter 3
Hormones and Puberty

Principles

Puberty Is a Rite of Passage!

Puberty, the acquisition of secondary sexual characteristics with the goal of attaining reproductive potential, marks an important portion of a developing adolescent's life journey. More than an event, puberty can span several years and not be associated with a clear 'terminal or climactic' ending. Puberty is also often plagued by 'starts' and 'stops' without clearly following a linear pattern in most adolescents; the progression of an individual's pubertal changes is determined by both genetic and environmental factors.

The adolescent will certainly be puzzled by some of the changes slowly altering the internal and external state of their bodies. Reassurance about the normalcy of these changes, ideally long before they first appear, both in the home and clinical setting, is essential.

The series of changes brought about during puberty are masterfully orchestrated by the hypothalamic pituitary gonadal (HPG) axis. The impulses released from the hypothalamus and the corresponding response from the pituitary start to increase in their amplitude and frequency, signaling to the ovaries in girls and the testicles in boys that it is time to begin the process of attaining secondary sexual characteristics. This process can begin as early as 8 years of age in girls and 9 years of age in boys. Over the last one to two decades, there has been a shift toward earlier onset of puberty, particularly in girls due to environmental factors such as increasing body mass index percentiles and access to higher caloric density nutrition.

A. J. Chattha et al., *Adolescent Medicine in the Middle East: Principles, Perspectives, Practices*, https://doi.org/10.1007/978-3-032-12348-0_3

In girls, the first sign of puberty mediated by the HPG axis is breast budding, also known as thelarche. Shortly thereafter, pubic and axillary hair development can occur, collectively known as adrenarche. Onset of adult-onset body odor and acne occur alongside these changes, signifying the rising hormone concentrations. There is often a growth spurt that occurs next, earlier in girls than boys, that is associated eventually with the onset of menstruation in girls. The average age at which menarche occurs is around 12 to 13 years of age, although geographical and ethnic variations occur.

For boys, pubertal signs are again initiated by the HPG axis and testicular enlargement occurs as a result. Through the course of ongoing puberty, enlargement of the genitals including the phallus occurs, followed by morning erections and emissions. A growth spurt tends to occur in the latter half of the pubertal years, allowing boys to typically attain a taller final adult height than girls, due to the higher number of years they spend in puberty.

Apart from attaining final adult height and reproductive capability, puberty is also related to bone mass accrual for both boys and girls, such that bone density or strength in adulthood is strongly predicted by the pubertal pace and hormone concentrations. Any disorders of pubertal development can therefore impact final adult height, reproductive potential and/or bone density.

The HPG Axis—Master Conductor of Puberty
The Hypothalamic-Pituitary-Gonadal (HPG) axis is the central command center for puberty. It's a complex interplay where the hypothalamus signals the pituitary, which in turn signals the ovaries or testicles, initiating the cascade of hormonal changes that define pubertal development.

Khadija Ali Alola, MD
Manama, Bahrain

Early Puberty

Pubertal signs and symptoms that signify true centrally mediated changes through the HPG axis are breast or testicle enlargement in girls and boys, respectively. If these changes occur prior to age 8 years in girls or 9 years in boys, they can signify an aberration in the course of puberty.

The causes of early or precocious puberty in both boys and girls can be divided into central disorders where the HPG axis is affected or peripheral disorders where the gonads (ovaries and testicles) are producing pubertal levels of hormones earlier than normal.

Centrally mediated early or precocious puberty can be due to any stressor, injury, genetic mutations or even space occupying lesions affecting the HPG axis. In girls, the cause of early puberty of central origin is unknown or idiopathic in greater than 80% of cases. If true evidence of premature puberty occurs in boys, it is more concerning due to the higher likelihood of finding a central pathology.

Causes of early puberty due to higher production of sex hormones can be ovarian cysts and rare tumors. Adrenal disorders such as congenital adrenal hyperplasia and genetic syndromes such as McCune-Albright syndrome can also cause early puberty. The common reproductive health disease known as polycystic ovary syndrome (PCOS) has also been associated with early development of pubertal characteristics, although it is unknown if the premature pubertal development leads to a PCOS type phenotype or vice versa.

More recently, endocrine disruptors or chemicals that may alter the course of puberty have been identified in household products, diets, and even medications. These can also lead to changes in the timing and sequence of puberty.

Once menstruation occurs in girls, it may take two to three years to have monthly menstrual bleeding due to ongoing immaturity of the HPG axis. For girls, abnormalities in flow and duration of the menstrual period as well as dysmenorrhea may be important considerations to address.

Late Puberty

For girls, delayed puberty is diagnosed if there is absence of secondary sexual characteristics by 13 years of age or lack of a menstrual period by age 15, a condition also referred to as primary amenorrhea. In boys, lack of secondary sexual characteristics by 14 years of age defines delayed puberty.

The causes of delayed puberty in adolescents can again be divided into those occurring centrally and affecting the HPG axis as well as those directly affecting the ovaries and testicles.

In the causes of centrally mediated delayed puberty, constitutional delay of growth and puberty where there is a family history of delayed growth is the most common cause. Malnutrition, chronic illnesses such as inflammatory bowel disease, head trauma, tumors, or stressors can also cause delayed puberty through the central axis. Particularly in adolescent females, eating disorders or unhealthy relationships with food can be a common cause of delayed puberty or lack of menstrual periods.

For conditions directly affecting the ovaries and testicles, genetic syndromes such as Turner syndrome or Klinefelter syndrome, structural anomalies leading to absence of reproductive structures such as uterus and vagina, polycystic ovary syndrome (PCOS), which may be associated with either early puberty as well as delayed menarche, post chemotherapy/irradiation damage to gonads or autoimmune disorders can be causes.

Early Puberty: A Shifting Timeline
Over the last two decades, there's been a noticeable trend towards earlier pubertal onset, especially in girls. Factors like increasing body mass index (BMI) and access to calorie-dense nutrition are believed to contribute to this shift.

Khadija Ali Alola, MD
Manama, Bahrain

Menstrual Disorders

The burden of menstrually related disorders in adolescent females is staggering. According to a recent study, almost all (97.8%) adolescents endorse at least one menstrually related disorder. These can range from menstrual irregularity, often considered within the realm of normal in the first few years post menarche to severe symptoms of premenstrual syndrome (PMS), being classified as premenstrual dysphoric disorder (PMDD). In addition to these, heavy flow, frequent leak through accidents causing stress and embarrassment particularly in school settings, severe pain during menstruation and intermenstrual bleeding are other common disorders of menstruation.

Common menstrual concerns can be divided into:

(a) Oligomenorrhea—a condition of abnormally infrequent menstrual periods such that the menstrual cycle is over 35 days long or there are less than 9 menstrual periods a year. From immaturity of the HPG axis to several disorders affecting the central nervous system as well as polycystic ovary syndrome, oligomenorrhea can have varied etiologies.

(b) Menorrhagia—defined by excessive or prolonged bleeding often requiring more than 5 menstrual products a day, frequent soiling of clothes, bleeding lasting for more than 7 days or associated with more than 80 cc of blood loss with periods; several pictorial blood assessment charts are used in the evaluation of menorrhagia. In adolescents, it is important to recognize that structural lesions such as polyps and fibroids occur less commonly than in adults. In an adolescent just presenting with menorrhagia, ruling out of the bleeding diatheses as well as hypothyroidism is essential. Pelvic ultrasound imaging may not always be warranted.

(c) Dysmenorrhea—this is painful menstruation, typically associated with cramping or sharp pain in the lower pelvis without any laterality. It can be primary in which case no organic pathology is identified and it is thought to be due to production of prostaglandin during menstruation leading to cramping. Secondary dysmenorrhea is less common in adolescents and could be attributed to endometriosis or pelvic inflammatory disease.

(d) PMS and PMDD—premenstrual symptoms, when they become severe enough to affect quality of life, sleep and appetite, can be classified as premenstrual dysphoric disorder or PMDD. These bring about a significant reduction in quality of life and inhibit functioning. Assessment is typically performed via detailed interview and questionnaire completion.

Polycystic Ovary Syndrome

The rise in obesity and sedentary lifestyle of many adolescents has also fueled an increase in states of insulin resistance. One such condition that can affect up to 4% of adolescents is Polycystic Ovary Syndrome (PCOS). The prevalence of PCOS is increasing around the world, including in the Middle East. The rising prevalence of PCOS is attributed to changing lifestyle and dietary choices, in addition to genetic predisposition. PCOS has important short-term cosmetic implications on skin and hair including but not limited to acne, unwanted hair growth called hirsutism, as well as darkening on the neck and in axillae known as acanthosis nigricans. In addition, long term complications of diabetes and thickening of the blood lining of the uterus, termed endometrial hyperplasia, may also occur. PCOS can adversely impact fertility, particularly if untreated. Last but not the least, several mood disorders such as anxiety, depression, sleep, sexual dysfunction, and eating disorders have a higher prevalence in adolescents with PCOS, even after accounting for their weight/BMI and socioeconomic factors.

To fulfill the diagnostic criteria of PCOS based on Rotterdam classification, an adolescent must exhibit 2 out of the following 3 conditions:

1. Symptoms of oligo/anovulation—typically manifesting as menstrual irregularity beyond the first one to two years after menarche or presenting as delayed menarche despite acquisition of secondary sexual characteristics.
2. Clinical or biochemical evidence of hyperandrogenism—androgen concentrations in the upper range of normal for the references established by a specific laboratory are sufficient to make a diagnosis in the appropriate clinical setting.
3. Polycystic ovarian morphology on ultrasound—either ovary with a volume greater than 10 cc may meet criteria for polycystic ovarian morphology in adolescents. Since adolescents typically do not consent to a transvaginal ultrasound, transabdominal imaging of the ovaries does not allow counting of follicles, limiting the application of adult criteria based on follicle numbers of PCOS in the adolescent setting.

Perspectives from the Middle East

Puberty

Ethnic and geographic variations strongly determine the onset, pace and sequence of pubertal changes. Puberty brings forth a myriad of emotions, and it is the role of the pediatrician, family medicine or adolescent medicine clinician to guide the adolescent through the throes of puberty. Concepts should revolve around reducing pathology, particularly with minor delays or changes in pubertal patterns. Modeling compassion, empathy and grace to the adolescent during this period of physical and emotional change, so they can hopefully extend the same to themselves, is critical. Physical signs of puberty such as adult type body odor and acne can be particularly challenging for the teenager to be forthcoming to discuss. An astute provider can offer many opportunities to begin these conversations and guide a review of hygiene measures as well as first line treatments for acne. These conversations should ideally precede the development of secondary sexual characteristics. Sensitivity in imparting this knowledge is necessary so the clinician does not inadvertently pathologize some aspect of puberty that the adolescent may be comfortable with such as acne. It is better to ask open ended questions such as *'are you thinking about any of the changes of puberty and having difficulty coping with any of them?'* instead of *'we can talk about acne and its treatment today,'* especially if the adolescent has not touched on that subject herself or himself.

Disorders of Puberty

Similarly, conversations around diet and physical activity are also important to have in a sensitive manner. As research suggests, empathic conversations regarding weight gain and a sedentary lifestyle can be effective change drivers. Yet, the same conversation had in an abrupt manner or even seemingly placing blame on the adolescent can be detrimental. While the long-term implications of pubertal disorders, particularly PCOS and the risks of development of PCOS, are important to consider and discuss, sensitivity in these subjects is crucial. Ineffective weight management counseling can be a trigger for disordered eating. Adding elements of motivational interviewing such as open-ended questions is particularly helpful for adolescents. For example, questions such as "how is your current weight affecting your life?" or "are there any reasons you would want to bring about a change in your body weight?" Waiting on a response, no matter how long it takes the adolescent to formulate one, is important. Establishing goals, together, and engaging a team is likely to lead to higher success rates with weight management.

In the Middle East, where rising trends of obesity and overweight have led to a steady increase in rates of type 2 diabetes and cardiovascular disease, it is also important to consider the cultural influence of food here as a harbinger of success, abundance, and social connections and community. Obesity can be multifactorial and, to a certain extent, beyond the control of the adolescent, due to the emphasis on large social gatherings, typically revolving around sprawling spreads of food. In certain cultures in this part of the world, being overweight may also be associated with a "plentiful blessings" mind set. To further complicate the discussion of weight management, opportunities for physical activity due to the hot climate, particularly outdoors, may be limited. Most indoor gym opportunities would involve travel to an appropriate facility, further limiting its access to those adolescents who are highly motivated.

Boys may have questions about final adult height and their growth potential as they lag behind their female peers through early puberty. This is particularly important in the Middle East where a recent review of growth hormone prescription practices has revealed that growth hormone is often prescribed in the setting of idiopathic short stature. Several of these individuals may have genetic short stature but with the use of growth hormone therapy have possibly attained a higher final adult height than would have been predicted based on genetic potential alone. Final adult height is typically an important aspect of discussion with adolescents in the Middle East, along with the parents. Requests may be made by family for additional evaluation and consultations with a pediatric endocrinologist if height potential is not being realized to the satisfaction of the patient and family.

These conversations regarding final adult height should also be dealt with in a sensitive manner and confidentially, if the adolescent desires.

Due to the Middle Eastern society being conservative in its outlook towards sexual and reproductive health discussions, conversation surrounding changes of puberty may not have been had at home. Therefore, the pediatrician, family medicine clinician or adolescent medicine practitioner is ideally positioned to broach the subject and to dispel myths (Figure). Confidential interview use, where possible with the adolescent patients, both female and male, can help establish a relationship with the healthcare provider that can unearth important health concerns.

Depending on conversations regarding changes of puberty that adolescents may or may not have had at home, their minds might be preoccupied by some of the changes in their physical appearance as well as the morning erections and emissions. Pediatricians should provide a safe space and begin anticipatory guidance in the prepubertal years to limit distress and increase association of positive attitudes to these changes. If the adolescent recalls a conversation with their clinician wherein it was discussed that these changes are normal, expected, and about to start shortly, the sense of well-being associated with these changes increases.

Similarly for girls, particularly in cultures where conversations regarding menstrual hygiene may not be forthcoming and open, the pediatrician is perfectly poised to impart education regarding menstrual hygiene products and expectations around menstruation well in advance. Several products for menstrual hygiene that have recently become available such as menstrual period underwear may not be easily accessible; therefore, imparting knowledge about these options, particularly in the Middle East, where tampons are less likely to be used for fear of disrupting the hymen, is important.

Both early onset menarche and delayed menarche can bring unique fears to the minds of adolescent girls and their parents. Fertility is an extremely important aspect of overall health, particularly in this community, and reassurance regarding the expected normal outcomes of most menstrual disorders in females, even if they presented with an early or late menarche, should be incorporated in the discussion with both the adolescent and the parents.

Similarly, experiences of PMS, or its more severe counterpart PMDD, may be challenging for the adolescent to bring up on her own. Open-ended questions focusing primarily on mental health before and during menstruation can help normalize some of the emotions experienced. *"How do you feel around the time your menstruation is about to begin?"* *"Do you feel your emotions vary between the days leading up to your menstrual period, while you are menstruating, and right after?"*

Including the adolescent in any discussion regarding treatment options they have utilized as coping mechanisms for PMS and PMDD increases compliance with additional suggestions made by the clinician.

Understanding of the "normal" aspects of the degree of blood loss during menstruation, as well as the appropriate amount of cramping to expect due to prostaglandin production, may also be limited. Establishing menstrual periods as excessively heavy or painful, based on a thorough history and log of symptoms, is important in order to review treatment strategies. There is hesitation on the part of adolescents in the Middle East as well as on the part of their families to begin hormonal therapy for menstrual management. It is often associated with the perception of interfering with ideal fertility potential. Dispelling these myths and reviewing safe, long-term options for menstrual management in adolescents paves the way for a smooth transition from childhood to adolescence and eventually to adulthood.

Although the low-dose, long-acting, reversible contraceptives that contain only progesterone, such as the arm implant which has a duration of action of three years or the intrauterine device which can last anywhere from five to eight years, are now widely available in other areas of the world, access to these devices and their use remains limited in the Middle East at this time. Particularly with regard to the intrauterine device insertion, even if it is to be done under sedation, there may be fear in the minds of several families following the Islamic faith that the hymen is likely to be disrupted in the process.

Although PCOS is increasing in its prevalence along with obesity rates in the Middle East, several misconceptions regarding its pathogenesis and eventual long-term implications exist. There are several unique aspects of care for PCOS in the Middle East. Since much of the counseling regarding PCOS involves dietary interventions, referring to the sensitivities and nuances reviewed above in the weight management section are important. Cosmetic implications, particularly if not brought up by the adolescent, can be inquired about an open-ended fashion since medication may be available to treat this. From the perspective of long-term complications, discussion of any impact on fertility must be carefully weighed. Thankfully, early diagnosis in adolescents coupled with appropriate weight management significantly reduces fertility impact from PCOS, and this information can be shared with families. This may provide not only reassurance but also added motivation to continue to work on lifestyle changes. As mentioned above, there may be hesitation in using hormonal management and a compromise may need to be reached regarding intermittent use of hormonal management to allow withdrawal bleeds at least once every three months to reduce risks of endometrial hyperplasia in PCOS. Intermittent use of progesterone-only pills for ten days every three months if there is amenorrhea in the interim, is often more acceptable to families in the Middle East than a daily hormone method.

Practices in the Middle Least

Puberty

Adolescent medicine clinicians are uniquely poised to provide sensitive and well-timed information regarding pubertal changes. At every annual health visit, depending on age and maturity of the child, physical examination for sexual maturity rating or Tanner staging, should be completed and anticipatory guidance given. Same gender providers can evaluate adolescents and, as good practice, always include a chaperone with the examination. Obtaining consent from the adolescent patient prior to proceeding with any confidential interview or sensitive physical examinations is vital.

Disorders of Puberty

Height and weight assessments and discussion of body mass index can be included with every physical examination. Instead of focusing on one point on the growth chart, the trajectory of the growth should be evaluated. If there are increasing BMI percentiles, focus on dietary changes and physical activity can delay or prevent onset of important secondary health complications such as PCOS, type 2 diabetes and cardiovascular disease. Screening with fasting glucose, hemoglobin A1c, a fasting lipid panel, and AST and ALT as a limited liver disease panel to rule out nonalcoholic steatohepatitis can be employed in both boys and girls where the BMI has crossed the 85th percentile.

Similarly, any discussion of pubertal changes including breast development, acne, or adult type body odor can be conducted with or without the presence of family members, taking direction from the adolescent. Some of these discussions, while they may be uncomfortable, can be very valuable for an adolescent. Open-ended questions focusing on body image, reaction and coping with pubertal changes, mood, and relationships with peers are important to consider each year, or sooner when there are specific concerns.

With pubertal changes will come many opportunities to identify aberrations in development. Therefore, if a child is early or delayed in attaining certain pubertal milestones, investigations including laboratory measurements of hormone, bone age and possibly ultrasound of the pelvis can be considered. Since puberty is inherently related to fertility, reassurance during this process of investigation is key, particularly in the Middle East where these conversations are a topic of significant concern and sensitivity. Families may also want additional reassurance that no 'invasive' physical examinations involving the pelvis will be performed, in order not to disrupt the hymenal membranes. The pediatrician should take every step possible to be accommodating of these requests. Most evaluation for early or delayed puberty can be completed with the use of a transabdominal pelvic ultrasound which would not involve transvaginal probing. The adolescent may also request any investigations that assesses impact on fertility be kept confidential from extended family members due to implications on future relationships. Confidentiality and maintenance of privacy are essential in every healthcare setting but are particular important in the Middle Eastern community.

Early Puberty

Essential investigations for early puberty in females after obtaining a detailed personal and family history including mid-parental height calculation, may include a bone age, transabdominal pelvic ultrasound, LH, FSH, estradiol, TSH, free T4, and prolactin measurements. Based on presence of hirsutism or increase in BMI, total and free testosterone, dehydroxyepiandrostenedione sulphate (DHEA-S) or 17-hydroxy progesterone (17-OHP) to rule out adrenal pathology can also be obtained. If there is concern for a centrally mediated process leading to early development of pubertal signs and symptoms, imaging of the brain including focus on the pituitary gland with an MRI may be warranted. Pituitary hormone profiles including IGF-1 and IGF BP3 and cortisol measurements may also assess the pituitary axis. In rare cases, particularly if there is a familial pattern or dysmorphism identified on examination, genetic testing may also be requested. With the exception of estradiol measurements or pelvic ultrasound, similar evaluation can also be obtained for males presenting with early signs of pubertal development.

Delayed Puberty

Evaluation for delayed pubertal development can include baseline testing including bone age which is a wrist x-ray in those over 3 years of age, complete blood count, comprehensive metabolic panel, TSH, free T4, estradiol (females), celiac disease testing if warranted, total testosterone (males), LH, FSH, prolactin, and genetic evaluation if warranted. Pelvic ultrasound imaging in females can be considered if there is lack of onset of menstrual period by 15 years of age or three years following the development of secondary sexual characteristics.

Beyond Reproduction: Puberty's Role in Bone Health
Puberty is not just about growth and reproductive potential. It is also a critical period for bone mass accrual. The pace of pubertal development and hormone concentrations significantly predict adult bone density and strength, highlighting the long-term impact of pubertal health.

Khadija Ali Alola, MD
Manama, Bahrain

PMS and PMDD

Disorders of menstruation including PMS and PMDD involve the use of mood stabilizing medications and antidepressants such as selective serotonin reuptake inhibitors (SSRI) as a first-line therapy. Along with this, counseling services are also very important. Hormonal methods for menstrual management such as oral contraceptive pills or progesterone-only pills or devices can also be considered for mood stabilization. Keeping an adequate log of symptoms as a means of determining when the severity of these disruptions in mood become most prominent can help guide treatment. There may be stigma associated with discussion and diagnosis of mental health disorders. As with other counseling with adolescents, sensitive sharing of information with only the adolescent and close family members is important. Pledging complete confidentiality and privacy of information can also ease their minds.

Menstrual Disorders: More Common than Realized
Nearly all (97.8%) adolescent females experience at least one menstrually related disorder, ranging from irregular periods to severe premenstrual symptoms. This underscores the importance of open discussions and appropriate management for these conditions.

Khadija Ali Alola, MD
Manama, Bahrain

Dysmenorrhea and Menorrhagia

Dysmenorrhea and menorrhagia can bring about significant disruptions in quality of life. Addressing these impacts with the use of validated questionnaires such as Period ImPact and Pain Assessment (PIPPA) and the Adolescent Menstrual Bleeding Questionnaire (aMBQ) can quantify baseline impairment, and repeat assessments using the same questionnaires can measure the impact of interventions. Of note, questionnaires used to identify heavy menstrual bleeding in adults may not be accurate for adolescents. Both dysmenorrhea and menorrhagia can be addressed with the use of non-hormonal and hormonal methods. Often, adolescents and their families would like to begin with non-hormonal interventions. Since the primary cause for dysmenorrhea in young teenagers is associated with prostaglandin secretion, scheduled use of non-steroidal anti-inflammatory drugs such as ibuprofen during the first two to three days of menstruation can be quite beneficial in both reducing cramping and also in reducing the amount and duration of bleeding. Use of tranexamic acid at a dose of 1300 mg three times daily for the first five days of menstruation is synergetic with ibuprofen in its impact on reducing bleeding and subsequently dysmenorrhea. If after three to six months of non-hormonal therapy, quality of life remains impacted by dysmenorrhea and menorrhagia, hormonal methods such as oral contraceptive pills, patches or long-acting, progesterone-only, low-dose devices such as the implant or intrauterine device, depending on its availability in the local area, can be considered. A baseline pelvic ultrasound may be obtained if dysmenorrhea and menorrhagia is severe but, often, these are primary diagnoses in adolescents without there being concurrent structural pathologies to rule out. It is important to obtain a bleeding diatheses panel along with a blood type, when the adolescent is *not* on hormone therapy, in those with very heavy menstrual bleeding along with epistaxis, easy bruising, or other signs of excessive bleeding. Thyroid dysfunction, particularly hypothyroidism, is also important to exclude in the evaluation of menorrhagia.

Polycystic Ovary Syndrome

The evaluation of possible polycystic ovary syndrome includes a thorough history and determination of frequency of menstrual bleeding. Primary or secondary amenorrhea as well as oligomenorrhea can be presenting signs of polycystic ovary syndrome. The diagnosis becomes more likely in the setting of acne, acanthosis, and/or hirsutism. Male pattern baldness or voice change may also be present in more severe cases. In order to rule out mimickers of PCOS such as adrenal tumors or congenital adrenal hyperplasia, evaluation with serum DHEA-S and 17-hydroxyprogesterone, respectively, is vital. When this evaluation is being obtained, total and free testosterone and occasionally androstenedione, which is a purely ovarian androgen, can be helpful in the diagnosis of PCOS. PCOS evaluation also involves exclusion of other hormonal disorders which is why thyroid function testing, LH, FSH, estradiol, and prolactin evaluation is also important at the time the androgen levels are being obtained. Ultrasound is not essential in making a diagnosis of PCOS in adolescents but can be obtained if the androgen testing is equivocal.

Treatment of polycystic ovary syndrome does involve consideration of lifestyle factors that can increase the risks of insulin resistance and type 2 diabetes. Involving a dietitian as well as a weight management team early in the course of treatment of PCOS is associated with higher chances of reversal of weight gain. Metformin therapy and the newer GLP-1 agonists can both be utilized in PCOS for weight management, in addition to and not as a replacement of physical activity. Aerobic activity for 30–60 minutes daily that consistently raises the heart rate of the adolescent is good aerobic activity for patients with PCOS that mitigates the risk of additional metabolic disorders.

Prevention of endometrial hyperplasia with PCOS involves hormone therapy. As mentioned above, there may be hesitation and myths or fears surrounding this treatment. Intermittent progesterone-only pill therapy can be employed in order to avoid amenorrhea for longer than 3 months at a time.

Early attention to disordered eating, sleep, sexual function and mood disorders such as depression and anxiety is also important in PCOS. Higher rates of mental health disorders have been noted in PCOS, beyond what would be expected based on weight or BMI. Reassurance regarding likely normal outcomes for reproductive ability, particularly with early diagnosis and attention to lifestyle changes, can be given. Having a low threshold for initiation of selective serotonin reuptake inhibitor (SSRI) treatment, thought to be the gold standard in treatment of mood disorders in PCOS, is reasonable.

Yearly evaluation for metabolic dysfunction including fasting glucose, hemoglobin A1c, lipid panel, and liver enzyme testing is important. There is a role for oral glucose tolerance testing as the goal standard of diagnosis of insulin resistance in PCOS is an impaired glucose tolerance but compliance may be a concern. If there is risk of the adolescent not returning for another stand-alone appointment for the glucose tolerance test, it is acceptable practice to obtain fasting glucose and hemoglobin A1c levels. Studies have evaluated a combination of random glucose testing with a hemoglobin A1c as also being predictive of metabolic dysfunction. Since adolescents are often heavily involved in school and activities, completing any essential testing at the time they are seen for the visit instead of scheduling for another date that they may not be able to attend, can be good practice in selective situations.

Pediatricians can review the need for and safety/efficacy profiles of all the hormone treatment options if a child with dysmenorrhea, menorrhagia, or PCOS requires one of these. It can be stressed that there is no impact on long-term cancer risk or fertility with the options used in adolescents while, in fact, *not* treating some of these conditions can have consequences on future health and fertility.

PCOS and Mental Health: An Overlooked Connection
Adolescents with Polycystic Ovary Syndrome (PCOS) have a higher prevalence of mood disorders such as anxiety and depression, even when accounting for weight and socioeconomic factors. This highlights the need for comprehensive care that addresses both physical and mental well-being in PCOS patients.

Khadija Ali Alola, MD
Manama, Bahrain

Hormone Therapy in Adolescents: Myths vs Facts

Fertility Myths

❌ Hormone therapy harms future fertility

✔ Does not reduce long-term fertility; may regulate cycles

Age Myths

❌ Too young for hormone treatment

✔ Safe and effective for teens when prescribed by a clinician

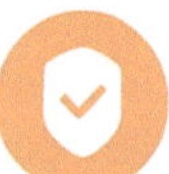

Safety Myths

❌ Hormone therapy is unsafe for adolescents

✔ Treatments are well-studied, carefully monitored, and individualized

❌ Natural remedies are always safer

✔ Many lack regulation or testing: medical therapies are standardized

Lifestyle/Social Concerns

❌ Hormones "mask" the real problem

✔ They can manage heavy bleeding, pain, and irregular cycles while underlying causes are evaluated

Hormone therapy in adolescents: myths vs facts

For Reflection

In your setting as you deal with adolescent girls with concerns about reproductive health, how can you best balance confidential care for adolescents emerging toward independent adulthood with a desire to keep parents fully informed and engaged?

Further Reading

1. Odongo E, Byamugisha J, Ajeani J, Mukisa J. Prevalence and effects of menstrual disorders on quality of life of female undergraduate students in Makerere University College of health sciences, a cross-sectional survey. BMC Womens Health. 2023;23(1):152. https://doi.org/10.1186/s12905-023-02290-7.
2. Al Jneibi SS, Taha F, Hammouri M, Allami Z, Weber S, Aljubeh J, Al Remeithi S. Recombinant growth hormone therapy in children with short stature in Abu Dhabi: a cross-sectional study of indications and treatment outcomes. Front Pediatr. 2025;13:1516967. https://doi.org/10.3389/fped.2025.1516967.
3. Biggs WS, Romeu JM, Gaudard T. Premenstrual syndrome and premenstrual dysphoric disorder: common questions and answers. Am Fam Physician. 2025;111(4):345–50.
4. Diaz A, Ayala Castro L, Carrillo-Iregui A. Short stature for the general pediatrician. Pediatr Rev. 2025;46(6):304–16. https://doi.org/10.1542/pir.2024-006538.
5. Trent M, Gordon CM. Diagnosis and Management of Polycystic Ovary Syndrome in adolescents. Pediatrics. 2020;145(Suppl 2):S210–8. https://doi.org/10.1542/peds.2019-2056J.
6. Özcan H, Burger NB, Dulmen-den Broeder EV, van Baal MW, den Boogaard EV, De Leeuw RA, Huirne JAF. Instruments to identify menstrual complaints and their impact on adolescents: a systematic review. J Pediatr Adolesc Gynecol. 2024;37(2):106–20. https://doi.org/10.1016/j.jpag.2023.11.011.
7. Al Mulla A, Lotfi G, Khamis AH. Prevalence of dysmenorrhea among female adolescents in Dubai: a cross-sectional study. Open J Obstet Gynecol. 2022;12(8):686–705. https://doi.org/10.4236/ojog.2022.128061.
8. Thannickal A, Brutocao C, Alsawas M, Morrow A, Zaiem F, Murad MH, Javed Chattha A. Eating, sleeping and sexual function disorders in women with polycystic ovary syndrome (PCOS): a systematic review and meta-analysis. Clin Endocrinol. 2020;92(4):338–49. https://doi.org/10.1111/cen.14153.

Chapter 4
Problems of Nutrition and Growth

Introduction/Overview

Worldwide and in the Middle East, between a third and half of adolescents have compromised nutrition and growth. Altered adolescent nutrition carries risks of immediate and life-long adverse health consequences.

Overweight and obesity are common in the Middle East, affecting about a third of most population groups studied. The prevalence of obesity has increased in recent decades and rose even more sharply during the COVID-19 pandemic.

Some adolescents simply do not eat enough, even though the underlying issues are often far from simple. This includes individuals who have eating-related symptoms (whether related to un-treated celiac disease or eosinophilic esophagitis or dysmotility or some other medical issue) that prompt them for comfort's sake to restrict their intake—a condition known as avoidant restrictive food intake disorder (ARFID). Some athletes become so focused on success in sporting activities that they neglect proper energy intake and develop resulting hormonal, skeletal, and systemic problems—a problem previously identified mostly in girls as the female athlete triad and now known as relative energy deficiency in sport (RED-S). Other adolescents develop altered perception of body image and then intentionally lose excessive amounts of weight with a variety of forms of eating disorders (EDs) including anorexia nervosa and bulimia.

Some adolescents, with or without overall adequate caloric intake, have inadequate intake of specific micronutrients. Vitamin D deficiency affects a third or more of adolescents in the Middle East, and iron deficiency is similarly prevalent. Patients with anorexia might develop thiamine deficiency, and older children and adolescents with autism spectrum disorder might restrict their intake in ways that lead to deficiencies of vitamin C and/or copper and/or other micronutrients.

A. J. Chattha et al., *Adolescent Medicine in the Middle East: Principles, Perspectives, Practices*, https://doi.org/10.1007/978-3-032-12348-0_4

Other seemingly healthy adolescents are shorter than they and their family would like. Related to cultural factors in the Middle East, concerns about short stature are raised more for boys than for girls.

Thus, several issues related to nutrition and growth are very common in the Middle East. In this section of *Adolescent Medicine in the Middle East* we review overweight and obesity, eating disorders, short stature, and two major micronutrient deficiencies.

Obesity

Approximately one-third of adolescents in the Middle East are overweight or obese. They have current consequences affecting blood sugar, liver health, sleep quality, and activity tolerance because of their weight. They are also at risk of life-threatening future consequences of obesity, including strokes and hypertension and early death. Overweight and obesity are important!

Principles

Overweight and Obesity Are Common and Identifiable

Obesity was common before the COVID pandemic with 15–20% of adolescents in the Gulf Countries of the Middle East overweight (body mass index, BMI, 85th to 95th percentile for age) and an additional 15–20% obese (BMI > 95th percentile for age). Overweight and obesity are even more common now! Changes in social contact and lifestyle and activity during the pandemic led to many more children and adolescents gaining excessive weight. A country's wealth is associated with its prevalence of obesity, and the risk of obesity rises with economic development.

> **Food Availability**
> Multiple 24/7 food delivery platforms and a vast variety of fast-food restaurants' availability have contributed to the increased prevalence of overweight and obesity.
>
> Yusur Turky Al Karaghouli, MBBS
> Abu Dhabi, United Arab Emirates

How do we define overweight and obesity? As suggested above, we calculate the body mass index. The BMI is the weight in kilograms divided by the height (in meters) squared. (Online calculators will do the calculation for you, such as at www.

nhlbi.nih.gov/health/educational/lose_wt/BMI/bmi-m.htm.) For individuals still growing longitudinally, it is good to present the BMI as its population-related percentile for the individual's age. These population determinations are based on what was normal in healthy populations about 25 years ago. BMI is not a perfect tool, but it is a reasonable screening test. Adolescents above the 85th percentile for BMI are considered overweight and should be identified, evaluated and, potentially, offered helpful treatment regimens. Adolescents at the 95th percentile or higher are considered obese and definitely should receive further evaluation and care.

Obesity Is Usually the Result of Multiple Factors Beyond the Adolescent's Control

Obesity is multifactorial. Many of the factors causing and exacerbating obesity have their origins long before the adolescent years. Even though part of the treatment will involve behavioral change of eating less and exercising more, we should be careful to avoid shame and guilt by hinting in any way that the obesity is the fault of the adolescent.

Back in the day, we figured that problems are caused either by nature (genetics) *or* nurture (upbringing). Certainly, genetic factors influence obesity. Overweight parents tend to have overweight children, whether due to genetics and/or upbringing. In addition, nurture, or parental behavior during a child's early years, also results in some children being trained to over-eat by rewarding good behavior with food or providing food as comfort from difficulties; this promotes over-eating and obesity by the adolescent years. Prenatal maternal BMI and parental eating behaviors are all associated with pediatric obesity. Nature *and* nurture both contribute to subsequent adolescent weight problems.

However, nature and nurture are not the only causes of adolescent obesity. Epigenetic factors also make a difference. Parents who suffered from food insecurity or starvation prior to becoming parents alter their epigenetic structures in ways that helps them better utilize limited food sources. Their children, then subsequently receive the same epigenetic influences and also are more likely to over-use their caloric intake, even if food is not scarce for them.

We also now know that the intestinal microbiome influences obesity. The variations of intestinal flora by presumed non-pathogens alters fat metabolism and other digestive processes which can lead to pathologic obesity.

Nature, nurture, epigenetics, and intestinal microbiomes. There are many factors beyond an adolescent's control contributing to excessive weight gain.

There are also other environmental factors that promote obesity. The way food is made available around the home and the family style of food consumption are two factors. In addition, lifestyle choices also matter. Some children choose, with the influence of their upbringing, to exercise more or less. Some families incorporate physical activity into daily lives more than do other families. Some families also incorporate eating into car rides and screen time in ways that foster over-consumption.

Thus, by the time, a child is an adolescent and able to make more independent decisions, the child is often already overweight or obese. Hormonal influences of normal puberty can then aggravate the problem.

A good understanding of the multifactorial nature of overweight and obesity reminds us not to blame or shame adolescents for their weight condition. Rather, we can focus on shared positive goals.

Overweight and Obesity Are Treatable, But Treatment Is Not Easy

Weight gain and weight loss are determined by a balance of caloric energy ingested on one hand and energy expenditure on the other. Eating more calories than needed to support physical activity results in weight gain; eating fewer calories than needed to support energy use results in weight loss. Thus, the "eat less and exercise more" approach to weight management is technically true.

But, weight management is not that straightforward. Beyond intake and use, there are other factors influencing the weight balance. Intake is partially managed by self-control, but psychological factors, whether stress or a desire for comfort food, also alter appetite and intake. Chemicals such as leptin can increase appetite, especially when sleep is altered or disordered. Then, intake is followed by absorption and metabolism; net intake can also be complicated by unusual losses (whether with unabsorbed sugars from the gastrointestinal tract with lactose intolerance, unabsorbed nutrients from the gastrointestinal tract with celiac disease or even diarrheal diseases, or sugar from the urinary tract with diabetes). Then, the nutrition that is ingested and absorbed must be either stored or used, and the storage depends on genetic and environmental factors. Metabolism varies between individuals related to genetics, hormonal balances, stress, and activity. The effects of physical activity on energy use also vary between individuals, related to size, genetics, and basal metabolic rate.

Thus, it is true that treatment of obesity depends on reducing caloric intake and increasing energy use. At the same time, however, effective treatment will also need to consider underlying treatable issues related to environmental factors, psychological make-up, concurrent illnesses, sleep habits, hormonal variations, and actual exercise.

> **Identify Triggers of Over-Eating**
> The key to helping an adolescent with reducing caloric intake is pinpointing the trigger(s) that cause their overeating (or occasional binge eating) and addressing them. These triggers could include boredom, loneliness, anxiety, stress, distractions, and mindless eating, among others. A technique frequently used to limit intake is practicing mindful eating; always keeping track of and identifying the body's cues to hunger and satiety.
>
> Yusur Turky Al Karaghouli, MBBS
> Abu Dhabi, United Arab Emirates

Medications, When Combined with Lifestyle Modification, Can Be Very Helpful

Historically, medications were not very effective in facilitating weight loss. Appetite suppressants, some of them with stimulant properties, could only briefly reduce intake, and there were concerns about side effects. Inhibitors of lipid breakdown could slightly reduce weight gain, perhaps even with a loss of 1–2 BMI points. However, these medications did not make major clinical differences.

Metformin has been effective in facilitating weight loss, especially in patients with polycystic ovary syndrome or type 2 diabetes. Loss of 2–3 BMI points could be expected.

Glucagon-like peptide-1 (GLP-1) receptor agonists such as semaglutide and liraglutide have revolutionized the medical management of obesity during recent years. GLP-1 receptors act in the brain to reduce appetite, in the pancreas to increase satiety and reduce food cravings, and on the stomach to prompt improved control of intake; these multiple effects promote reduced eating and, thus, weight loss. Regular injections were required, but oral agents are becoming available. A loss of about 15 kg (perhaps 5–6 BMI points) can be anticipated during the first year of treatment, and, with ongoing treatment, the weight is not re-gained.

Medications require ongoing treatment. At the same time, reduced intake and increased activity through lifestyle interventions are also needed to prevent a re-gaining of lost weight.

Surgery Holds Promise for Long-Standing Treatment Success

Several different surgical procedures have been used to facilitate weight loss, including gastric bypass and gastric size reduction through sleeves or bands; each is similarly effective. These procedures have typically been reserved for adolescents with severe obesity and medical complications of obesity (such as sleep apnea, steatohepatitis, and type 2 diabetes). However, weight loss is typically significant (up to 15 BMI points) and persistent. Statistically, surgery is a good option for overweight adolescents.

In Fact, the Obesity Epidemic Is, in Large Matter, a Consequence of Adolescent Lives Being out of Balance

Obesity is a problem. Widespread obesity is also a consequence of many other primary problematic features of adolescent society being out of balance. Obesity would become less common if societies were able to effectively promote: (1) appropriately healthy diets, (2) daily physical activity for all adolescents, (3) regular sleep schedules with, for adolescents, about nine hours of sleep each night, (4) positive peer interactions that foster mutual maturation and development without demoralizing adolescents for individual differences, and, (5) implementation of good stress management techniques.

Perspectives from the Middle East

Epidemiologic studies from throughout Middle Eastern countries show high rates of adolescent obesity, and obesity is becoming more common. Sadly, as in other regions of the world, there are not yet success stories of countries or large population groups that have significantly reduced the growing rates of obesity.

Awareness of the prevalence of obesity and of the consequences of obesity is widespread. The values of healthy diets and health-promoting physical activity are also well-known. In the Middle East as elsewhere, however, good knowledge is not commonly translated into health-enhancing behaviors.

Sedentary lifestyles (and video gaming) are common in the Middle East, as elsewhere. Excessive screen time is common. Presumed quick fixes for obesity are more attractive, even though not possible, than long-term daily interventions (whether lifestyle modification or medication). For patients with access to GLP-1 receptor agonists, there is a popular tendency to use medication without necessary concurrent changes in choices about intake and exercise, and the notion of necessary long-term use of medication is not always accepted.

Practices in the Middle East

Do Something About Obesity!

With 30% of adolescents being overweight and/or obese, physicians have ample opportunity to greatly impact the future health of entire populations by focusing on daily activities and promoting healthy lifestyles and maintenance of appropriate body weights. Public health interventions should popularize appropriate dietary intake, daily physical activity, good sleep habits, enhanced social interactions, and stress management; these efforts can combine to target various factors behind the epidemic of obesity.

Weight Management Is Important for all Patients

All individual patients should be encouraged to implement healthy lifestyle choices—not just about diet and exercise but also about sleep, stress management, and social interactions. Every clinical encounter should include assessment of BMI. When a BMI is over the 85th percentile for age, evaluation for an underlying (even if unlikely) pathologic cause should be considered, and interventions that at least include lifestyle modifications should be considered.

Table 4.1 Key messages for adolescents with obesity

1.	It's not your fault. There were many factors, some beyond your control, that led to you gaining too much weight
2.	It is not just about your weight. Your weight is a marker of problems but the real issue is that your current and future quality of life is being hindered. We should target interventions more on improving health than on just reducing weight
3.	You need tangible, practical, realistic goals. Sure, "exercise more, eat less "is proper advice, but that is too simplified and almost never really works. Pick measurable targets about intake to restrict, exercise sessions, sleep habits, fun activities, and stress management
4.	Choose when, why, how, and what to eat. Usually this includes avoiding comfort foods and avoiding eating while reading, watching screens, driving, or walking
5.	Integrate fun physical activity into daily life
6.	Mobilize a team. We all need help doing difficult tasks. Get parents, friends, and professionals to help you improve your health
7.	Keep your mind healthy and focused on proper goals
8.	Medication can actually help
9.	Surgery should not just be a last resort. It is part of an integrated management plan for improving the health of overweight people

Avoid Shaming

Of course, being overweight or obese is not necessarily the fault of the adolescent. Clinicians should avoid all hints of shaming and guilting when discussing concerns about the patient's weight. Rather, the weight/BMI can be acknowledged with questions as to whether the adolescent is concerned and if the adolescent thinks there might be a treatable medical condition behind this. Clinicians' questions can make it clear that there are likely genetic and environmental factors behind the patients' weight issues and that not all of those factors are treatable. At the same time, the clinician and patient can, together, explore possible lifestyle changes that might mitigate some of the adverse effects of the underlying causes of the overweight condition. The Table 4.1 provides key messages that can be clearly communicated to overweight adolescents.

Keep the Weight Concerns in the Context of the Adolescent's Life

When weight screening identifies overweight or obesity during an acute visit for a separate concern, the clinician should be careful to deal with the primary concern and not to pressure the patient about the weight. However, recognizing that the weight is up, especially if there is no sign of a treatable underlying cause, a clinician and patient can likely identify one straightforward intervention (perhaps reducing the consumption of sugar-sweetened beverages or not combining screen time with eating time or taking a daily walk with a friend) to try before a subsequent visit a month later. This might help prepare the patient and provide some success, even before lengthier discussions about the weight.

Start with Practical Interventions

Sometimes, healthy behaviors can be implemented fairly easily. Consideration could be given toward: (1) limiting non-educational screen time to less than two hours per day, (2) scheduling at least nine hours of nightly sleep, (3) scheduling at least 30 minutes of physical activity each day, (4) avoiding second servings during meals, (5) avoiding all sugar-sweetened beverages, and, (6) eating only while sitting during meal times, not while walking or driving or reading or watching a screen. Many overweight patients can cure their weight condition simply by implementing three or four of these interventions. Of course, patients who are already obese often need additional interventions.

> **Stack Habits**
>
> Remember that stacking habits is powerful and valuable with adolescents. Associate or add one intervention to an existing habit and then follow it with other interventions, steadily and gradually. As such, these newly acquired habits become implemented and incorporated into the adolescent's daily routine.
>
> Yusur Turky Al Karaghouli, MBBS
> Abu Dhabi, United Arab Emirates

Look for Causes, Contributors, and Consequences of Obesity

During an initial evaluation that was arranged specifically to focus on obesity, a clinician can review the growth chart—often using it to demonstrate that the excessive weight started years ago in childhood and that it is not merely a consequence of any of the adolescent's recent lifestyle choices. Through history and screening exams, clinicians should look for evidence of treatable causes of obesity (such as hypothyroidism, adrenal excess, and depression). Clinicians can then seek evidence of treatable contributors to obesity (such as iron deficiency and poor sleep habits). Concurrently, one should evaluate for consequences of obesity, both to treat them and to use them to predict outcomes; this would include consequences of obesity such as obstructive sleep apnea, steatohepatitis, altered glucose metabolism (whether insulin resistance or actual type 2 diabetes), dyslipidemia, and menstrual irregularities. Identified co-morbid conditions should be treated.

Together, Set Appropriate Goals

It is important for a clinician and a patient to choose mutually acceptable goals. Focusing on primary weight goals is often not the best option. Rather, weight can be monitored while working toward teen-relevant life goals such as being able to participate more comfortably in physical education classes, fit in with peers at the beach, or feel better.

Engage a Team

Weight management is not an individual activity. The clinician and patient must involve the family. The family plays important roles in sharing healthy activities, encouraging success, and avoiding any hint of nagging about either the weight or temporary failures in meeting treatment goals. Beyond the clinician and patient and family, it is usually good to involve a dietitian—to give helpful practical advice but not to give any hint that the obesity is the fault of the patient's past dietary indiscretions; we also want the patient to focus more on healthy behaviors than on specific calorie counts. Often it helps to engage a psychologist on the care team—to help the patient gain tools to maintain motivation for long-term lifestyle changes and to deal with whatever stresses and social dysfunction might be aggravating dietary challenges. Of course, an endocrinologist or gynecologist can be involved when there are specific co-morbid conditions in those domains.

The primary clinician can help set goals and then follow progress, emphasizing successes with eating, exercising, sleeping, and socializing more than focusing on a numerical weight. The clinician should cheer for the patient more than prod the patient toward improving health.

With an Established Foundation of Lifestyle Intervention, Consider Medication and Surgery

If there is already obesity, especially with co-morbid conditions, and if there is no improvement after an initial month or two of intervention, then consideration of medical management is appropriate. Metformin can be considered, especially if there is insulin resistance or polycystic ovary syndrome. If that does not prove effective, semaglutide could be considered. Of course, medications should always be combined with foundational lifestyle interventions. Most experts reserve bariatric surgery for those with severe obesity persisting despite six months of good efforts at lifestyle and medication interventions; however, surgery is likely to become increasingly common due to its proven effectiveness.

For Reflection

Review Table 4.1. Which of these messages do you routinely communicate to overweight adolescents? Which messages will you choose to start communicating?

Disordered Eating and Eating Disorders

Introduction

Adolescent diets are often disorganized and disordered. Many adolescents skip morning meals. Others eat irregularly. Quickly consumed processed fast-food replaces calm family meals of nutritious foods. Most adolescents survive disordered eating. All adolescents would benefit from good eating behaviors and appropriate dietary intake. Sadly, some adolescents develop serious life-threatening eating disorders.

Principles

Regular Healthy Meals Are Integral to Good Physical and Social Health

Meal times are good for nutrition and for social interaction with family members and peers. At home, in school, and even out in malls with friends, meal times afford opportunities to grow in relationships and in social skills. At the same time, popular foods are not always nutritious, and physical health depends on appropriate intake.

While Obesity Is Common, Adolescent Girls Even More Commonly Think They Are Overweight

A global nutrition study revealed that twice as many adolescent girls thought they were overweight as were actually overweight. Yes, obesity is common, but a false perception of obesity is similarly common among adolescent girls. This frequent belief that one is overweight can serve as the basis of unnecessary dietary restriction, inappropriate weight loss, and eating disorders. Physicians should foster appropriate understanding of adolescents' size and health status.

Anorexia and Bulimia Are Fairly Well-Known, But There Are Other Important Disorders of Restrictive Eating as Well

Characterized as a medical condition since the mid-1800s and now affecting 1–3% of adolescent females in resource-rich countries (and less than 1% of boys), anorexia nervosa (or, simply, "anorexia") is a condition of intentional weight loss with altered body perception (inaccurate belief of being overweight even if starving and wasted), often severe eating-related anxiety, food-associated obsessions, amenorrhea, dizziness, and bradycardia. Many patients with anorexia over-exercise and induce their own vomiting. Management is challenging and requires a multi-disciplinary team and long-term follow-up to ensure restoration of appropriate weight and control of altered body perceptions and anxieties.

Bulimia (or "bulimia nervosa") shares many features with anorexia but is specifically characterized by binges of over-eating followed by extreme feelings of guilt or shame which trigger self-induced vomiting or other forms of purging. Features are similar to those of anorexia, but weight loss is usually less extreme.

Avoidant restrictive food intake disorder (ARFID) is characterized by intentionally restrictive food intake, often prompted by an attempt to relieve physical symptoms and often resulting in nutritional deficiencies and unhealthy weight loss. Unlike patients with anorexia nervosa, patients with ARFID have appropriate perceptions of their body habitus. However, physical discomfort (sometimes co-occurring with gastrointestinal dysmotility and disorders of gut-brain interaction) prompts restrictive eating which partially relieves the bothersome abdominal symptoms and then leads to inadequate nutritional intake and inappropriate weight loss. Treatment would be considered after management of inciting pathologies and involves restoration of appropriate intake and weight.

Historically, female athletes sometimes restricted intake either due to being "too busy" to eat or to avoid having to propel extra body weight during sports activities. These adolescents then went on to have irregular or absent menses, decreased bone density—often with stress fractures, and inadequate energy to support desired athletic performance. This condition was previously known as female athlete triad. Over time, boys also had similar problems, and other concurrent symptoms were recognized. Now, the condition of relative energy deficiency in sport (RED-S) is more commonly known. The key feature of RED-S is a lack of energy to perform as desired, and other key findings include reduced reproductive health (disrupted menses for girls, altered libido for boys), increased incidence of stress fractures, altered immunity with more frequent infections, dizziness, and altered mood. Weight loss is not a necessary component of the condition, and affected adolescents do not have altered body image. Treatment is restoration of adequate intake to maintain a normal weight *and* to restore reproductive health, bone density, immunity, circulation, and mental health. Fortunately, with adequate energy intake, health returns *and* athletic performance improves.

The COVID-19 Pandemic Exacerbated the Problem of Eating Disorders

During the COVID-19 pandemic there were marked increases in the incidence of new diagnoses of anorexia. Concurrently, patients with anorexia had worsened symptoms, with deterioration in physical and mental health. The causes of this worsening were likely multifactorial, relating to altered social support systems, reductions in routine medical care, and fears about the potential fate of the world.

Perspectives from the Middle East

Eating disorder patients in the Middle East seem similar to those living elsewhere. The majority of adolescents with eating disorders are girls, but some boys are affected. Some but not all patients have been competitive or had pre-existing anxieties. There is sometimes but not always a family hyper-awareness of health (diet and exercise and weight) prior to the onset of the eating disorder. Patients get focused on food and eating, and some develop obsessions and compulsions. Some patients exercise excessively, some self-induce vomiting, and some try to promote excessive urination or stooling.

Patients with eating disorders in the Middle East, as elsewhere, are not necessarily dishonest, but they perceive themselves and situations differently than do other people. Thus, they truly think they are overweight or "fat," even when they are excessively thin and malnourished. They might even perceive seemingly dishonest activities (vomiting or exercising or adding heavy objects to their pockets prior to being weighed) as helpfully manipulation of the situation to better align the findings and results with their own perception of reality.

As elsewhere, families of eating disorder patients in the Middle East are usually lovingly committed to their children. The adolescent with an eating disorder is often cleverly able to manipulate the parents into facilitating the adolescent's own altered perceptions and unhelpful behaviors.

Cultural Considerations in Meal Support
In many Middle Eastern households, caregiving and meal support often involve extended family. Including key family members in Family-Based Treatment sessions helps align strategies and reinforces shared responsibility, enhancing support and consistency during recovery.

Alanoud Al-Ansari, MD, MHPE
Doha, Qatar

Effective care of eating disorder patients requires an expert professional team. Unfortunately, pediatricians, adolescent medicine physicians, dietitians, and psychologists with experience in managing patients with eating disorders are not always available in all areas of the Middle East.

Practices in the Middle East

For All Adolescent Patients

As clinicians get to know patients and connect with them, it is reasonable to raise the topic of eating. We can ask about family meals and groups that eat together at school. We can ask about adolescents' outings for meals with friends. Our interest and our brief comments can validate and encourage healthy eating behaviors.

At the same time, we should notice growth parameters during all healthcare visits. We can pay particular attention to details about dietary restrictions. We would definitely pursue any items of concern with further questions or even with testing. Early diagnoses of feeding issues can lead more quickly to effective intervention.

Binging and purging are not uncommon in adolescents, and relevant questions can be included when completing a review of systems. Patients who binge and/or purge should be followed closely, with good discussions about maintaining appropriate body image and weight.

For Patients with Restricted Intake Without Body Image Concerns

Sometimes, we will realize that a patient before us is restricting foods. Even if the weight is adequate, we should seek symptoms and signs (and maybe even diagnostic testing) of food intolerances, allergies, malabsorption, dysmotility, and gastro-esophageal disease. Identified pathologies should be treated, but further evaluation would be needed if symptoms do not improve.

With non-judgmental open-ended questions, we should inquire about the adolescent's view of his or her body. Satisfied? Wanting to gain muscle mass? Feeling overweight? Of course, we would deal with identified pathologies. But, when there is restricted eating without evidence of body dysmorphic disorder, especially in the presence of weight loss, we should consider a diagnosis of ARFID. Education of the patient can be coupled with aggressive weight gain programs to restore health. Techniques of dietary management with ARFID is similar to treatments of patients with anorexia.

For an Athlete with Declining Performance and Health Changes

Secondary amenorrhea in an athlete is not part of normal health, and the addition of oral hormone supplements is not indicated. Stress fractures can result from over-training but can also be a sign of RED-S. If athletic performance is dropping, if there have been excessive infections, and if mood disorders are appearing, we should carefully focus on the timing of the symptoms and the details of dietary intake. It is likely that treatment with improved dietary intake will lead to improved athletic performance, stronger bones, reduced infections, and better mood. Dietitians can help guide nutritional intake, and actual weight gain is not always needed. At the same time, iron deficiency is common in athletes, and iron supplements can be provided to keep the ferritin level above 20 ng/dL. The goal of increased nutrition is to restore health (including regular menses, for girls) and performance, not necessarily to alter the weight. It is important to increase nutritional intake until healthy bodily functions are restored and maintained. Orthopedic colleagues can help plan a return to activity after fractures.

For Patients with Restricted Intake, Excessive Weight Loss, and Self-Perception of Being Overweight

Typically, adolescents with eating disorders present because the parents are concerned about restrictive eating or weight loss. Sometimes, the lack of menstruation will trigger medical care. The adolescent herself or himself rarely reports concerns or symptoms but might be seeking medical help to lose more weight or, if weight loss has already been dangerously excessive, might complain of dizziness and fainting.

Thus, it is important for the clinician, when seeing an adolescent with weight loss and/or amenorrhea and/or restrictive eating to seek details about previous weight measurements, daily dietary intake, exercise routines, and unusual vomiting or diarrhea. Open-ended discussion questions can help the clinician learn how the adolescent perceives her or his body and if the adolescent feels overweight or has a specific target weight. The patient's BMI percentile prior to the onset of weight loss is often a good target when planning therapeutic weight gain.

For patients with weight loss and a sense of still being overweight, clinicians must realize that the patient perceives the world differently than do healthy people. Thus, clinicians should not expect to develop a bonded, mutually agreeable relationship with eating disorder patients. Rather, the clinician must work with the family to ensure that the adolescent, willing or not, behaves in healthier ways. Eating is not an option about which the patient can decide; rather, the patient's decision might be limited to whether the nutrition goes in by eating or via nasogastric tube.

Most adolescents with anorexia become overly focused on weight and calories. It often helps *not* to let the patient be aware of her or his actual weight. It is also helpful to talk with the teen about restoring energy so that body systems work better rather than meeting specific caloric intake targets.

The most essential aspect of managing patients with anorexia is that of family-based therapy. If available, a skilled psychologist can implement family-based therapy; otherwise, this can be accomplished by primary clinicians, nurses, or social workers. Professionals engaging in family-based therapy empower the family to structure the patient's living situation so that healthy behaviors are implemented. It is the illness (anorexia) that controls the adolescent's intake; the patient is not in control of her or his eating. The disease is the problem, and neither the family nor the patient should sense personal guilt or shame for having the condition. Clinicians help families and patients focus on appropriate behaviors rather than discussing causes of the condition. Families and clinicians do not need to negotiate with the patient, but they must set up firm controls, limits, and behavior modification strategies. It is often difficult for parents to impose meals on a child, and it often helps if parents can enforce eating behaviors as a means to rewards and privileges that are desired by the patient; for instance, a patient who enjoys phone access might be awarded phone time only after complying with essential intake.

The 4 Cs of Meal Support
Supporting adolescents at mealtimes is a key part of eating disorder recovery. The 4 Cs of meal support: Calm, Confident, Clear, and Consistent help caregivers and clinicians create a steady, reassuring environment. Staying calm, trusting the plan, setting clear expectations and responding firmly and predictably can reduce anxiety and resistance, making mealtimes more manageable.

Alanoud Al-Ansari, MD, MHPE
Doha, Qatar

For patients with extreme weight loss or very low BMI (such as 13 or less) or symptoms such as dizziness, detailed evaluation is warranted. An electrocardiogram can rule out a significant dysrhythmia (beyond the usual mild bradycardia). Possible derangements of sodium, potassium, phosphorous, and magnesium should be evaluated. Comorbidities can be ruled out (or in) by testing for liver enzymes and thyroid function and iron deficiency.

Hospitalization is indicated if the heart rate is less than 50/minute, if there are other dysrhythmias on electrocardiogram, if there is symptomatic hypotension, if electrolyte levels are abnormal, and if the weight is not increasing despite aggressive outpatient treatment. In the hospital, the focus is on ensuring adequate nutritional intake—targeting a normal intake (not, as in previous years, starting with suboptimal intake and increasing gradually). Refeeding syndrome is possible when feeding normally after extreme weight loss, so electrolyte (with phosphorous and magnesium) testing once or twice daily is warranted for the initial period (often about two days) of re-feeding, with supplements provided as needed.

If the patient will not take in the targeted normal nutrition by mouth, nasogastric feeding is a reasonable option. Intravenous treatment would only be needed for the very short-term if there was persisting symptomatic hypotension. Careful discussion with the patient and family and care team is helpful in achieving compliance with nasogastric feedings.

As the weight rises to within a couple kilograms of the target (for height) weight, the patient usually becomes more compliant with treatment and has some reduction in self-destructive behaviors. Nonetheless, feeding will be required, observation is needed to prevent self-induced vomiting, and physical exercise should be limited until the weight is increasing regularly and the patient is taking in the desired oral intake. Feeding supplement formula is reasonable for short-term initiation of treatment, but the goal is to have the patient eating normal food with regular meals. When needed, hospitalization is usually only necessary for a week or so.

> **Understanding Emotional Challenges in Recovery**
> As weight restoration progresses in adolescents with eating disorders, psychological distress often increases. Many patients experience heightened anxiety, body image concerns or resistance to treatment during this phase. Normalizing these feelings as part of the recovery journey can help adolescents stay engaged in treatment.
>
> Alanoud Al-Ansari, MD, MHPE
> Doha, Qatar

Ongoing treatment success depends on good collaboration between the family, the primary physician, a dietitian, and a psychologist. Medication is not usually effective for anorexia, but some patients with extreme food-related anxieties and/or with eating-related obsessions and compulsions can be helped by medication managed by a psychiatrist. Medications used in this setting include second generation anti-psychotics (dopamine-serotonin antagonists such as quetiapine) and third generation anti-psychotics (dopamine partial agonists such as aripiprazole).

Most patients with eating disorders can get back to a desired weight and have good dietary intake within a few months. Nonetheless, the risk of recurrent symptoms remains, and long-term follow-up is needed for at least several years.

For Reflection

Many pediatricians are people-pleasers. We want our patients to like us. We want to communicate well with them and develop good working therapeutic relationships. This is almost always good and desirable—but not necessarily effective with patients with anorexia. Think about how you can communicate with an adolescent with anorexia and help the family set up appropriate behavioral limits even when the adolescent will disagree with your treatment plan.

Short Stature

Principles

Definition Short stature is a clinical term signifying a child whose height is substantially below the expected range for age, sex, and population. The most widely accepted definition is a height more than **2 standard deviations (SD) below the**

mean for the same age, sex, and population norms. Often, for ease of interpretation, clinicians would utilize the less than third or fifth percentiles as a threshold for decision making.

Height that falls below this threshold should always prompt an evaluation for potential growth-related concerns but the majority of children will be found to be healthy and these deviations will be a variant of normal.

Epidemiology and Prevalence in the Middle East

Short Stature Prevalence Varies widely across the Middle East, reflecting intricate interplays between genetics, nutrition, psychosocial factors, and healthcare access. For example, within Saudi Arabia, national surveys revealed significant regional differences with the southwest region reporting much higher prevalence of short stature in children and adolescents, approximately 18.8% compared to other regions where it is between 6.5 and 14%. This could reflect disparities in nutrition and socioeconomic status.

Particularly in areas affected by armed conflict and displacement, under-nutrition and its impact on children is quite evident. In these situations, rates of moderate to severe stunting are high. Lack of access to healthcare delivery further exacerbates problems in these regions.

Other Contributing Factors

Other factors also contribute to variations in the prevalence of short stature among differing populations. These factors include:

1. High rates of consanguinity leading to autosomal recessive disorders,
2. Large family sizes, delayed complementary feeding, and suboptimal weaning practices, and,
3. Urban-rural healthcare disparities.

Genetic Syndromes in Middle Eastern Populations

The Middle East is characterized by unique genetic epidemiology due to high rates of consanguinity, particularly in Saudi Arabia where rates of consanguinity can reach 58%, promoting expression of autosomal recessive disorders. Universal newborn screening may also not be readily available in all regions of the Middle East.

Cultural Factors Affecting Management

Cultural norms Play a Profound Role in the perception, detection, and management of short stature. Large, extended family structure can sometimes provide support but occasionally brings stigma, buffering or accentuating emotional difficulties. Religious beliefs may also impact attitudes towards genetic counseling, prenatal diagnosis, and acceptance of medical interventions. Misconceptions about normal growth and the value of medical evaluation persist.

Healthcare Access and Endocrine Services

Access to specialist pediatric endocrinology services is highly variable in the Middle East with urban centers generally having better availability than in rural areas. There may also be insurance-related and cost barriers for people in many regions in the Middle East.

Classification of Short Stature in Children

Physiologic Short Stature

Idiopathic short stature (ISS) denotes children with no identifiable cause for their short stature after thorough evaluation. Other categories include **familial short stature** (FSS), wherein a child is short but has short parents and a growth rate consistent with their family background, and **constitutional delay of growth and puberty (CDGP)**, characterized by delayed physical maturation and a lower growth velocity that can normalize eventually after a later growth spurt.

Pathologic Short Stature

In contrast to the above, **pathologic short stature** may result from a wide range of genetic, psychosocial, endocrine, nutritional, and systemic disorders. Early recognition and management of these pathologic conditions can profoundly influence final adult height and overall health.

Growth Charts and Normative Data

Growth Chart assessment can vary widely by country. Typically, in the Middle East, World Health Organization (WHO) growth chart standards are recommended, reflecting optimal growth patterns for children up to 2 years of age and Centers for Disease Control and Prevention (CDC) growth chart norms for those between 2 and

20 years of age. There have been more recent growth charts devised that are reflective of local population data that are starting to be utilized in Saudi Arabia and UAE.

These charts plot height, weight, and body mass index (BMI) with percentile curves determined statistically from populations of healthy children.

The concept of **mid-parental height** is essential in growth assessment. It estimates a child's genetic potential, with the following formulas:

- For boys: [(father's height + mother's height) + 13 cm] ÷ 2
- For girls: [(father's height—13 cm) + mother's height] ÷ 2

A projected adult height within 2 SD (~10 cm) of the mid-parental height strongly suggests normal familial growth variation.

Key Points in Growth Monitoring

- Serial plotting of height reveals **growth velocity**, a sensitive marker for growth disorders.
- **Crossing downwards of percentiles** over time is more concerning for underlying pathology than simply being consistently short.
- Disease-specific and ethnicity-specific growth charts are available and may be necessary for certain conditions (e.g., Turner syndrome, Trisomy 21/Down syndrome)

Genetic Etiologies of Short Stature

Genetic factors are the most important determinant of final adult height, with heritability estimates exceeding 80%. However, there is a complex interplay between genes and environmental modifiers.

Familial Short Stature (FSS) has traditionally been seen as a normal variant but there may be an underlying monogenic, often autosomal dominant, disorder leading to subtle forms of growth plate dysplasia or hormone pathway defects that can be inherited in families. (See Table 4.2) In these cases, there may be several family members that are relatively short. Recently, whole exome sequencing (WES) has been able to uncover many of these genetic causes of short stature.

Endocrine Causes of Short Stature

Table 4.3 lists common causes of short stature and with the appropriate diagnostic evaluation can often lead to effective treatment and reversal of the delayed/reduced growth. Normal or, at least, improved adult height can be achieved.

Table 4.2 Key monogenic genetic causes and associated clinical features

Genetic cause/ syndrome	Associated Genes	Clinical features
SHOX gene deficiency	SHOX	Seen in Leri-Weill dyschondrosteosis and Turner syndrome; 2–15% of short stature cases; variable phenotype
Noonan syndrome & RASopathies	PTPN11, SOS1, RAF1, others	Short stature, distinct facial features, congenital heart defects, delayed puberty
ACAN gene mutations	ACAN	Advanced bone age, short stature, possible early-onset arthritis
FGFR3 mutations	FGFR3	Achondroplasia and hypochondroplasia; disproportionate or proportionate short stature
Collagenopathies	COL2A1, COL11A1, other	Mild disproportionate short stature, subtle, syndromic features
Other genetic syndromes	Various (e.g., Turner 45,X, trisomy 21, etc.)	Includes Turner syndrome, Down syndrome, Silver-Russell, Prader–Willi, and others

Table 4.3 Endocrine cause of the short stature and associated diagnostic clues

Endocrine cause	Key features	Diagnostic clues
Growth hormone deficiency (GHD)	Poor growth velocity, increased weight, delayed bone age, hypoglycemia, midline anomalies	Stimulation testing, low IGF-1/ IGFBP-3 levels
Hypothyroidism	Decelerated growth, delayed bone age, constipation, fatigue, dry skin	Newborn screening (for congenital), clinical signs (acquired)
Cushing syndrome	Suppressed linear growth, preserved weight	History of steroid use or signs of cortisol excess
Delayed or absent puberty	Impaired pubertal growth spurt, adolescent onset	Clinical evaluation of pubertal development
Other hormonal deficiencies	Signs of pituitary dysfunction, possible CPHD	Hormonal assays (TSH, ACTH, gonadotropins), pituitary imaging

Nutritional Causes of Short Stature

Protein-energy malnutrition and micronutrient deficiencies can profoundly affect final adult height. Such deficiencies include those of iron, zinc, and vitamin-D, particularly in resource-limited settings, but also in affluent societies due to selective eating, chronic illness, or eating disorders.

Malabsorption occurring from chronic gastrointestinal disorders such as celiac disease and inflammatory bowel disease can also cause poor absorption of nutrients resulting in stunting and wasting. Children born small for gestational age (SGA) can generally achieve catch-up growth within the first two years of life, but persistent short stature beyond this period can signify inadequate nutrition or an underlying genetic disorder.

Psychosocial Factors Influencing Growth

Psychosocial Short Stature (PSS) (also called "psychosocial dwarfism") is a rare disorder resulting from extreme emotional deprivation or chronic stress that can present anywhere between two and 15 years of age and is characterized by:

1. Profound short stature and low weight,
2. Inappropriate skeletal age (delayed bone age), and,
3. Unresponsiveness to intended nutritional intake, as stress suppresses endogenous growth hormone secretion.

Children affected by severe, protracted familial or institutional neglect, abuse, and violence such as is seen in areas of war and armed conflict may exhibit stunted growth due to a disrupted stress axis. Timely removal from the adverse circumstances can restore normal hormone levels and result in catch-up growth.

Less extreme circumstances of chronic stress such as bullying in school or difficulties can also lead to internalization of symptoms and some impact on mental health as well as diminished growth velocity.

Perspectives from the Middle East

Unique aspects of short stature evaluation in the Middle East require focus on genetic, endocrine, nutritional, and psychosocial aspects of the child and his or her community.

Genetics

The high rates of consanguinity, expectations of marrying within one's own tribal community and large family sizes in many Middle Eastern populations contribute to a higher prevalence of autosomal recessive disorders and clustering of rare genetic syndromes. This can impact the phenotypic spectrum and prevalence of short stature due to genetic causes in the region.

Whole exome sequencing (WES) is increasingly available throughout the Middle East, although such testing is not universal. Genetic testing is increasingly being employed to understand genetic etiologies of short stature, particularly in families.

Endocrine Evaluation

Newborn screening for endocrine disorders is increasingly widespread in Middle Eastern countries, with some exceptions. However, after a diagnosis is made, coverage and access to advanced diagnostic and therapeutic modalities remain geographically variable.

Nutritional Aspects

Regional disparities in short stature prevalence closely mirror socioeconomic disparities. In several Middle Eastern countries, stunting remains common, especially among marginalized groups, rural communities, and in the context of chronic conflict and displacement.

Psychosocial Risks

While the common extended family structure in Middle Eastern societies may buffer some psychosocial distress, it can also lead to delayed detection in reporting of mental health concerns due to considerations regarding family honor and stigma associated with psychological disorders.

Practices in the Middle East

Clinical Diagnostic Approach: History and Physical Exam

Key Elements of the Clinical Approach

1. Detailed History:

- Prenatal factors: maternal health, birthweight/length, gestational age, complications.
- Family history: parental heights, history of delayed puberty, consanguinity, known genetic disorders.
- Nutritional history: feeding patterns, appetite, dietary restrictions, food insecurity.
- Chronic diseases: symptoms suggestive of chronic illness or systemic disease.
- Social environment: history of psychological stress, trauma, or neglect, exposure to armed conflict and displacement.

2. Physical Examination:

- Anthropometric measurements: accurate height, weight, body proportions, BMI.
- Serial measurements: plotted on appropriate growth charts.
- Pubertal staging: Tanner staging for sexual maturation.
- Physical features: dysmorphic features, disproportion, limb abnormalities, midline defects.
- Signs of underlying disease: chronic illness indicators, organomegaly, skin, hair, and nails.
- Signs of psychological distress: Hygiene, upkeep of clothing/hair, signs of trauma from conflict or displacement

3. **Growth Velocity Assessment:**

- Serial height measurements every three to six months (ideally over six to 12 months), to document growth velocity.

Children showing **reduced growth velocity**, deviation from their genetic potential, or loss of upward percentile trajectory require further evaluation.

Clinical Diagnostic Approach: Laboratory Investigations

Laboratory and Ancillary Testing can be tailored to the underlying clinical findings although basic laboratory evaluation may be indicated in all those who presents with short stature.

Recommended Initial Investigations:

Complete blood count (CBC), ESR, CRP
Comprehensive metabolic panel
Thyroid function (TSH, free T4)
Celiac serology (tTG-IgA and Total IgA)
IGF-1 and IGFBP-3
Karyotype (phenotypic girls)
Urinalysis
Additional tests, as indicated by clinical findings

Growth hormone stimulation testing is reserved for those with clinical signs or laboratory evidence suggestive of growth hormone deficiency (GHD), as random growth hormone levels are not reliable due to pulsatile secretion.

Genetic Testing (targeted or exome sequencing) is warranted if initial workup is unrevealing or if clinical features suggest a syndromic disorder.

Clinical Diagnostic Approach: Imaging and Bone Age

Bone Age Assessment via Radiograph of the Left Hand and Wrist is a very useful adjunct to the clinical examination. The most widely used standard is the **Greulich and Pyle atlas** method, comparing the patient's radiograph to reference images by age and sex.

Bone Age Interpretation
- **Delayed bone age** often indicates constitutional delay or an endocrine disorder (GHD, hypothyroidism).
- **Bone age concordant with chronological age** is typical in familial or idiopathic short stature.
- **Advanced bone age** suggests states of androgen or estrogen excess as well as some genetic disorders.

Imaging may also include:

- **MRI of the hypothalamic-pituitary region**: indicated for confirmed GHD or clinical signs suggestive of midline central nervous system pathology (such as micropenis and midline craniofacial defects).

Management of Short Stature

Management of short stature varies based on the specific, identified cause of short stature.

Growth Hormone Therapy Guidelines

Growth Hormone Therapy (rhGH) is the mainstay of treatment for selected causes of short stature. Approval and initiation of therapy may take time and involve paperwork to obtain funding.

- Growth hormone deficiency
- Turner syndrome
- Noonan syndrome
- Prader-Willi syndrome
- Chronic renal insufficiency
- Children born small for gestational age without catch-up growth by age 2
- SHOX deficiency
- Idiopathic short stature (ISS), with strict criteria

Therapy is generally administered as daily subcutaneous injections. Newer long-acting formulations (weekly injections, such as somatrogon and lonapegsomatropin) are now commercially available in some regions of the Middle East. However, these are not universally available. Longer-acting formulations can improve compliance with the treatment regimen.

Typical Criteria for Initiation and Monitoring
- Confirmation of the specific diagnosis by a pediatric endocrinologist.
- Regular monitoring of growth response (height velocity), IGF-1 levels, and side effects.
- Annual reassessment for efficacy and side effects.
- Dose adjustments based on body weight, growth response, side effects, and laboratory parameters.

Outcomes and Expectations
- Children with GHD: marked improvement in height, often reaching within normal adult range if diagnosed and treated early.
- Turner syndrome/SHOX deficiency: significant gains of 5–10 cm in final height expected.

- Idiopathic Short Stature: modest height gains (3–7 cm as compared to untreated peers); cost-effectiveness and risk-benefit are debated.

Safety

rhGH has a robust safety record when used appropriately, with most side effects (edema, mild hypothyroidism, headaches, joint pain) being mild and reversible. The possibility of rare serious events (e.g., benign intracranial hypertension, slipped capital femoral epiphysis, impaired glucose tolerance) should prompt regular monitoring.

Nutritional and Lifestyle Interventions

For children and adolescents whose short stature is due to nutritional deprivation or chronic illness:

- **Nutritional rehabilitation** is paramount, addressing both caloric intake and micronutrient supplementation.
- Behavioral feeding interventions, social support, and sometimes supplemental feeds are needed in more severe or refractory cases.
- Correction of underlying malabsorption (e.g., celiac disease via gluten-free diet) or systemic disorders will restore normal growth if managed early.

For most children with non-pathological (variant) short stature, there is **no evidence that special diets, vitamins, or supplements will improve height** if weight gain is normal.

Psychosocial Support and Counseling

The **psychosocial impact of short stature** varies. Issues include:

- **Bullying and stigma**, especially in peer and school environments.
- **Low self-esteem**, social withdrawal, and anxiety or depressive symptoms.
- **Performance and academic pressures** due to being misperceived as younger or less mature.

Interventions

- **Early psychosocial support** (counseling, peer support, family psychoeducation) is essential, especially for children with low self-esteem
- School-based accommodations and awareness can reduce bullying and misunderstanding.
- **Cultural sensitivity** is crucial in Middle Eastern contexts, where stigma or reluctance to seek mental health care are significant barriers.

International and Regional Guidelines

Guidelines for Short Stature Evaluation and Management are issued by global authorities such as the Pediatric Endocrine Society, Growth Hormone Research Society, American Academy of Pediatrics, National Institute for Health and Care Excellence (NICE), and regional organizations.

Key recommendations include:

- Use of appropriate growth charts (WHO for <2 years, CDC for $\geq$2 years).
- Prompt referral for children with height < -2 SD, poor growth velocity, signs of systemic illness, or variance from mid-parental height.
- Systematic approach—history, physical, laboratory, and imaging assessment.
- Consideration of genetic testing in idiopathic and familial cases, given high diagnostic yield in selected patients.
- GH therapy restricted to approved indications, with regular monitoring for efficacy and safety.
- Integration of psychosocial assessment as well as nutritional rehabilitation and support into all diagnostic and treatment pathways.

Regional Modifications are increasingly advocated to address local genetic, nutritional, and healthcare system nuances. In the Gulf and wider Middle East regions, there are growing rates of adoption of national screening programs, inclusion of premarital genetic counseling, and public health efforts targeting consanguinity and nutrition.

Conclusion

Short stature in children and adolescents is often multifactorial with genetic, endocrine, nutritional, psychosocial, and systemic etiologies. The Middle East presents unique patterns due to higher rates of consanguinity, nutritional disparity, and evolving healthcare systems. Rigorous application of algorithmic evaluation and evidence-based interventions is important.

- **Early diagnosis** and intervention, particularly in endocrine and nutritional causes, can normalize growth trajectories.
- **Genetic evaluation** is increasingly critical, especially in consanguineous populations and idiopathic/familial cases.
- **Growth hormone therapy** may be helpful for some indications and lead to a robust response in final adult height
- **Nutritional and systemic disease management** is foundational, while psychosocial intervention is often overlooked but is essential.
- **Cultural competence, healthcare access, and health system strengthening** are imperative for Middle Eastern reasons to ensure health access equity.

For Reflection

An 11-year-old boy is shorter than most of his peers. He has a completely normal evaluation with no sign of pathology. You believe he has familial short stature. The parents insist on providing growth hormone so he will grow taller. What ethical principles can guide your discussions with the parents and your treatment of the child?

Micronutrient Deficiencies: Vitamin D and Iron

Two specific micronutrient deficiencies are common in adolescents throughout the Middle Eastern countries. About half of adolescents are low on vitamin D, and nearly a third of girls and 10% of boys lack adequate iron.

Principles

Vitamin D Is Available

Vitamin D is found in only low levels in natural foods. Dairy products are often fortified with vitamin D, and sunshine stimulates a cutaneous reaction to produce vitamin D. Thus, adolescents require either sun exposure (equivalent to that of having the face and arms exposed to sunshine for about 20 minutes per day) or fortified beverages and foods to achieve adequate vitamin D status.

Vitamin D Deficiency Is Common

Around the world, vitamin D deficiency is common, especially in colder areas where skin is not exposed to sunshine during much of the year but also in the Middle East where hot weather precludes outdoor activity and cultural habits often leave most of the skin covered. Since vitamin D is stored in adipose tissue, overweight and obese adolescents tend to have lower circulating levels of 25-hydroxyvitamin D (the metabolite measured in the blood to determine vitamin D status) and to be more prone to the adverse effects of vitamin D deficiency.

Vitamin D Deficiency Is Associated with Serious Health Problems

Infants and young children can develop rickets from vitamin D deficiency, but that problem is limited to young children with rapidly mineralizing bones. Adolescents with vitamin D deficiency can reduce their peak bone density and mass and, thus, limit their adult bone density and strength. Hypovitaminosis D in adolescents is also associated, though causality is not proven, with later development of some cancers, immune deficiencies, and neurologic disorders such as multiple sclerosis.

Vitamin D Deficiency Can Be Prevented by Food Fortification, Medical Supplementation, and Sunshine Exposure

Ingestion of vitamin D fortified foods and beverages is effective in preventing vitamin D deficiency. Milk is the most commonly fortified product, but adolescents don't always consume much milk. Supplementation is recommended and, when used, effective to prevent vitamin D deficiency in infants and young children, but ongoing supplementation into and through adolescence is not routine. Sunshine exposure is totally effective in preventing vitamin D deficiency, but comfort and culture leave many adolescents, especially girls, with inadequate sun exposure. Thus, the effective means to prevent vitamin D deficiency are not routinely applied to adolescents in the Middle East.

Treatment of Suspected or Proven Hypovitaminosis D Is Effective in Restoring Normal Vitamin D Status, Yet Many Adolescents Remain Undiagnosed and Untreated

For infants and young children, vitamin D supplementation is routinely recommended in order to prevent nutritional rickets. Testing of vitamin D status in asymptomatic children is not necessary in view of managing current bone disease. However, for adolescents, there is not a consensus about whether to apply a *test and treat* strategy or a *supplement all* strategy in areas of the Middle East where vitamin D deficiency is common. Without consensus, many adolescents at risk of vitamin D deficiency are neither identified by screening tests nor supplemented; thus, vitamin D deficiency continues to be common even though supplementation is very effective at a dose averaging about 1000 IU/day. Since vitamin D is stored in adipose cells and persists in the body, administration can either be divided into daily or weekly or monthly doses.

Iron Deficiency Is Common and Consequential during Adolescence

Testing in many adolescent population groups in many areas reveals that approximately 30% of adolescent girls and 10% of adolescent boys are iron deficient. (The loss of iron-rich blood during monthly menstruation makes iron deficiency more common in girls than in boys.) Iron deficiency is causally associated with decreased academic performance, decreased exercise tolerance, and, when severe, anemia and cardiac dysfunction.

There Are Several Tests for Iron Deficiency, But the Ferritin Level Is the Most Useful

Iron deficiency can lead to microcytic hypochromic anemia, but iron deficiency alone is problematic even in the absence of anemia. Serum iron levels fluctuate widely over time but are sometimes low with iron deficiency. Limited (<14%) saturation of iron binding capacity is also suggestive of iron deficiency. The most sensitive and specific test for iron deficiency is the ferritin level since it indicates iron storage. (Of note, however, the ferritin level may be normal or elevated when there is inflammation present along with iron deficiency.) Typically, a ferritin level of at least 20 ng/mL is considered adequate, though some experts prefer that a ferritin level be maintained at 50 ng/mL or more (especially if there are learning concerns or sleep disorders present). Measurement of the soluble transferrin receptor is an excellent test for iron deficiency (with high levels indicating iron deficiency) and is not subject to false positivity in the presence of inflammation, but this test is not widely available.

Iron Therapy Is Effective

Iron therapy must be continued until iron stores are repleted *and* the cause of iron deficiency has been corrected (whether excessive blood loss from menstruation, inadequate iron absorption due to untreated celiac disease, or limited iron content in the diet). Typically, oral iron therapy should be continued for three or more months. Intravenous iron allows a single dose of iron to provide for three weeks of treatment, but the risks and cost of intravenous infusions coupled with the need for longer-term oral supplementation leave intravenous iron limited to only the most severe cases.

The dose of iron supplementation to treat deficiency is usually 3–5 mg/kg/day. Traditional teaching has been to divide the total daily dose into three separate administrations each day, preferably on an empty stomach and with concurrent administration of vitamin C to facilitate iron absorption. This frequent between-meal dosing is not easy for adolescents, and many teens report abdominal discomfort or constipation with treatment. At the same time, recent research indicates that hepcidin levels rise with each iron dose given and that higher hepcidin levels inhibit iron absorption—making it seem that daily or every other day dosing should be adequate.

Perspectives from the Middle East

Children who look healthy and report no symptoms can still be deficient in vitamin D and/or iron. This is true in both wealthy and impoverished populations in the Middle East. Thus, clinicians should have a low index of suspicion for these micronutrient deficiencies. And, when it is known that the local prevalences of these deficiencies are high, one should consider routine supplementation with vitamin D and routine advice about iron-rich foods. When vitamin D supplementation is not accepted and/or when diets are not rich in iron, testing could be done to confirm deficiency and to encourage appropriate corrective intervention.

Vitamin D Deficiency—Lessons from Recent Research
A retrospective study analyzing vitamin D levels over five years in Saudi Arabia* found persistent high prevalence (>60%) of deficiency with minimal year-on-year improvement despite awareness campaigns. This implies that preventive measures are inadequate and reinforces the need for routine supplementation or fortification strategies.

Vanitha A Jagannath, MBBS, MD
Manama, Bahrain

*www.frontiersin.org/journals/public-health/articles/10.3389/fpubh.2025.1535980

Studies in most Middle Eastern countries show that 30–80% of adolescent females (and nearly as many males) are vitamin D deficient. Widespread supplementation would be sensible; lacking that, individual testing and treatment would be recommended.

Vitamin D Deficiency—Specific Issues in the Middle East
Despite ample year-round sunlight, vitamin D deficiency is highly prevalent (30–80%) among adolescents of both genders. Cultural clothing practices and limited outdoor activity due to heat highlight the need for contextual supplementation strategies rather than reliance on sun exposure. As vitamin D is stored in adipose tissue, rising adolescent obesity rates in the Arabian Gulf region compound the situation, suggesting tailored dosing and preventive public health interventions.

Vanitha A Jagannath, MBBS, MD
Manama, Bahrain

Iron deficiency is common, yet compliance with iron supplementation is sometimes uncomfortable due to abdominal pain. Thus, testing of iron status (with a ferritin level at a time when the adolescent is not ill with an infection or an inflammatory condition) would be warranted as a routine screening measure; those with ferritin levels less than 20 ng/mL would be treated (with about 4 mg of elemental iron per kg of body weight in a single oral daily dose, even as the diet is enriched with iron-containing foods and menstruation, if heavy, might be treated medically).

> **Iron Deficiency Prevalent Even in High-Income Settings**
> Iron deficiency affects ~30% of adolescent girls and ~ 10% of boys, including those from wealthy urban populations. This underscores that micronutrient deficiencies are not limited to socioeconomic deprivation but also to dietary patterns (low meat intake, high refined carb diets) and menstrual losses in girls.
>
> Vanitha A Jagannath, MBBS, MD.
> Manama, Bahrain.

Practices in the Middle East

Interventions to correct micronutrient deficiencies in patients and populations flow directly from what has been discussed already in this chapter. But, it is important to keep interventions relevant to the local situation and context.

Vitamin D Deficiency

Practically, there are decisions to be made about screening versus targeted testing, dosing of supplementation and treatment, and follow-up evaluation.

In areas where more than 10 or 20% of adolescents have vitamin D deficiency, one option would be to supplement all adolescents with 600 to 1000 IU of vitamin D every day. (Or, a single weekly or monthly supplement could be given instead with the dose equaling what would be given with combined daily doses—4000 to 7000 IU weekly or 18,000 to 30,000 IU monthly.) Overweight and obese adolescents would be treated with doses at the higher side of the suggested range. Supplementation could continue for many years.

Sometimes, however, physicians or families might prefer only to supplement if deficiency has been confirmed. Generalized screening of all adolescents in high-risk areas could be instituted. Or, more targeted screening of higher-risk individuals could be implemented. If an adolescent has less than an hour each week of head and arm exposure to the sun, it would be reasonable to screen for vitamin D deficiency. If an adolescent has gastrointestinal symptoms suggestive of malabsorption (loose or smelly stools, abdominal bloating) or known celiac disease, it would be reasonable to screen for vitamin D deficiency. If an adolescent has chronic pain, screening for vitamin D deficiency is also reasonable. The threshold for screening would be lower in overweight and obese adolescents than in thin teens, and the testing threshold would be lower for individuals with more darkly pigmented skin.

The best screening test for vitamin D deficiency is the 25-hydroxyvitamin D level. Blood can be sampled at any time of day, without regard for recent food intake. Those with identified deficiency (level less than 50 nmol/L, which is the same as 20 ng/mL) should be supplemented with an average of 1000 IU of daily vitamin D. (Both vitamin D2 and vitamin D3 are similarly safe and effective.)

If follow-up testing is desired (such as when there is concern for adequate intestinal absorption of vitamin D), it could be done after a month of treatment. Achieving a normal level of 25-hydroxyvitamin D, however, is not an indication to stop treatment unless it is certain that the original problem causing vitamin D deficiency (whether inadequate sun exposure or malabsorption) has been corrected.

School-Based Sun Exposure Break

Even in sunny regions, vitamin D deficiency remains high due to limited outdoor activity. Structured sun breaks within school schedules can serve as an effective public health intervention to reduce deficiency rates without cost-intensive supplementation programs. Schools could implement a daily 20-minute outdoor break, perhaps during mid-morning or early afternoon when ultraviolet B light is adequate but heat is tolerable. Faces and forearms should be exposed. Hydration should be ensured.

Vanitha A Jagannath, MBBS, MD
Manama, Bahrain

Iron Deficiency

Iron deficiency should be suspected when an adolescent has excessive bleeding, when an adolescent has unexplained fatigue, and when there are sleep problems (especially with leg discomfort at the time of sleep onset, suggestive of restless leg syndrome). In addition, of course, iron deficiency should be considered when there is limited intake of meat. Especially for adolescent girls, one might consider routine screening for iron deficiency, even when the patient is asymptomatic. Sometimes iron testing would be considered as part of a general adolescent health maintenance visit.

Ferritin levels are the most useful, readily-available test for iron deficiency and are reflective of actual iron stores. Serum iron levels fluctuate with recent iron intake and are less predictive of an actual deficiency. Saturation of iron binding is a useful test, but still not as helpful as a ferritin level. However, ferritin levels are most useful when the patient is well since inflammation, even that associated with an acute febrile illness, can prompt elevations of ferritin levels even in the face of significant iron deficiency.

In an adolescent without signs of inflammation, a ferritin level of less than 20 ng/mL indicates iron deficiency, whether or not there are any other symptoms.

Some academic clinicians actually prefer to consider levels less than 25 or even 50 g/mL as being too low. Especially for adolescents with sleep disorders or neurologic disease, a level of at least 50 ng/mL is sometimes targeted.

Of course, iron deficiency is not a *primary* diagnosis. Once iron deficiency is identified, a clinician should seek to understand the cause. While dietary insufficiency of iron is a common cause of iron deficiency, other causes are possible—such as excessive menstrual blood loss or poor iron absorption due to celiac disease. Especially if iron deficiency is not easily resolved with supplementation, evaluation for blood loss and malabsorption should be considered. If excessive bleeding is suspected as the cause of iron deficiency, that, too, might not be the fundamental primary diagnosis; testing for coagulopathies including von Willebrand disease would be appropriate. Whatever underlying cause of iron deficiency is identified, treatment of that primary disorder would be helpful.

Possible School-Based Interventions

1. Dietary Iron Enrichment in Schools

   Integrate iron-rich meals and snacks into school canteen menus. Focus on fortified cereals, lean meats (beef, chicken), legumes, lentils, spinach, leafy greens, and iron-fortified breads or wraps. Pair these foods with vitamin D-rich foods such as oranges and Bell peppers to increase absorption. Couple the dietary changes with nutrition education sessions, parental involvement, and monitoring of meal uptake.

2. Menstrual Health Management for Iron Deficiency

   Integrate screening for heavy menstrual bleeding using history-based questionnaires into adolescent health curricula, ensuring personal confidentiality. Provide access to school nurses or linked clinics for evaluation.

   Facilitate referral pathways for medical management (e.g. hormonal therapy) when needed.

Vanitha A Jagannath, MBBS, MD
Manama, Bahrain

Typically, iron is given in a dose of 3 to 5 mg/kg/day. Oral dosing is best absorbed when given with vitamin C at a time when there is not another divalent cation such as calcium competing for absorption; thus, dosing is best on an empty stomach. Intravenous iron is only rarely needed, such as when there is severe symptomatic deficiency complicated by intestinal malabsorption of iron. Emerging data suggest that liposomal iron might be adequately effective with fewer side effects.

Recent studies of hepcidin have implications for the frequency of iron dosing. Hepcidin, when released from the liver, regulates bioactivity of iron. Iron intake prompts hepcidin release which leads to reduced intestinal absorption of iron. Thus, excessively frequent iron dosing could keep hepcidin levels elevated and reduce absorption of subsequent iron doses. Practically, this means that daily iron dosing might be better than divided doses (and is certainly easier). Adult studies suggesting limiting iron doses to every two or three days have not been replicated in adolescents. Thus, it is currently reasonable to give 3–5 mg/kg of elemental iron in a single daily dose for adolescents who have ferritin levels less than 20 ng/mL.

Therapeutic iron supplementation is necessary until iron stores are replenished (usually at least three months later) *and* the underlying condition has been corrected. If, for instance, dietary intake of iron or heavy menses have not been resolved, iron treatment might be needed for many months.

> **Limited Routine Supplementation Policies**
> Routine vitamin D or iron supplementation programs for adolescents are not universally implemented in Middle Eastern countries despite high prevalence.
>
> This gap offers scope for policy recommendations integrating supplementation into school health programs or adolescent wellness initiatives.
>
> Vanitha A Jagannath, MBBS, MD
> Manama, Bahrain

For Reflection
You realize that half of the adolescent girls tested for 25-hydroxyvitamin D in your area have low levels. As you and your colleagues discuss approaches to this problem, what factors will help you decide whether to: (1) ignore the problem since they are too old to develop rickets, (2) test all adolescents who come to you, (3) suggest school-based screening, and/or, (4) advocate for vitamin D supplementation of all adolescent girls in your area?

Further Reading

1. Zhang X, Liu J, Ni Y, Yi C, Fang Y, Ning Q, Shen B, Zhang K, Liu Y, Yang L, Li K, Liu Y, Huang R, Li Z. Global prevalence of overweight and obesity in children and adolescents: a systematic review and meta-analysis. JAMA Pediatr. 2024;178(8):800–13. https://doi.org/10.1001/jamapediatrics.2024.1576.
2. Liu C, Chow SM, Aris IM, Dabelea D, Neiderhiser JM, Leve LD, Blair C, Catellier DJ, Couzens L, Braun JM, Ferrara A, Aschner JL, Deoni SCL, Dunlop AL, Gern JE, Rivera-Spoljaric K, Hartert TV, Hershey GKK, Karagas MR, Kennedy EM, Karr CJ, Barrett ES, Zhao Q, Lester BM, Check JF, Helderman JB, O'Connor TG, Rasmussen JM, Stanford JB, Mihalopoulos NL, Wright RJ, Wright RO, Carroll KN, McEvoy CT, Breton CV, Trasande L, Weiss ST, Elliott AJ, Hockett CW, Ganiban JM, Environmental influences on Child Health Outcomes (ECHO). Early-Life Factors and Body Mass Index Trajectories Among Children in the ECHO Cohort. JAMA Netw Open. 2025;8(5):e2511835. https://doi.org/10.1001/jamanetworkopen.2025.11835.
3. Shanti Vaidya S, Taylor BM. Glucagon-like Peptide-1 agonists and pediatric obesity. Pediatr Rev. 2025;46(2):123–5. https://doi.org/10.1542/pir.2024-006455.

4. Stefater-Richards MA, Jhe G, Zhang YJ. GLP-1 receptor agonists in pediatric and adolescent obesity. Pediatrics. 2025;155(4):e2024068119. https://doi.org/10.1542/peds.2024-068119.

5. Ryder JR, Jenkins TM, Xie C, Courcoulas AP, Harmon CM, Helmrath MA, Sisley S, Michalsky MP, Brandt M, Inge TH. Ten-year outcomes after bariatric surgery in adolescents. N Engl J Med. 2024;391(17):1656–8. https://doi.org/10.1056/NEJMc2404054.

6. Attia E, Walsh BT. Eating disorders: a review. JAMA. 2025;333(14):1242–52. https://doi.org/10.1001/jama.2025.0132.

7. Alharbi Y, Saleh F, Shahat KA. Effective treatment approaches for eating disorders in children and adolescents: a review article. Cureus. 2024;16(11):e74003. https://doi.org/10.7759/cureus.74003.

8. Stoody VB, Garber AK, Miller CA, Bravender T. Advancements in inpatient medical Management of Malnutrition in children and adolescents with restrictive eating disorders. J Pediatr. 2023;260:113482. https://doi.org/10.1016/j.jpeds.2023.113482.

9. Fisher M, Zimmerman J, Bucher C, Yadlosky L. ARFID at 10 years: a review of medical, nutritional and psychological evaluation and management. Curr Gastroenterol Rep. 2023;25(12):421–9. https://doi.org/10.1007/s11894-023-00900-w.

10. Gould RJ, Ridout AJ, Newton JL. Relative energy deficiency in sport (RED-S) in adolescents – a practical review. Int J Sports Med. 2023;44(4):236–46. https://doi.org/10.1055/a-1947-3174.

11. Riss V, Hartman-Munick SM, Shubkin CD, Lahey T. A bitter pill: the ethics of involuntary treatment of adolescents with severe eating disorders. Hosp Pediatr. 2025;15(2):e66–72. https://doi.org/10.1542/hpeds.2024-007921.

12. Caro R, Savel P, Moss PI. Evaluation of short and tall stature in children. Am Fam Physician. 2025;111(6):532–42.

13. The Pediatric Endocrine Society. Short stature. 2020. https://pedsendo.org/patient-resource/short-stature

14. El Mouzan MI, Al Herbish AS, Al Salloum AA, Al Omer AA, Qurachi MM. Regional prevalence of short stature in Saudi school-age children and adolescents. Sci World J. 2012;2012:505709. https://doi.org/10.1100/2012/505709.

15. Yousef NA, AA EH, Shaik NA, Banaganapalli B, Al Ghamdi AF, Galal AH, Alahmadi TS, Shuaib T, Aljeaid D, Alshaer DS, Almutadares M, Elango R. Nationwide survey on awareness of consanguinity and genetic diseases in Saudi Arabia: challenges and potential solutions to reduce the National Healthcare Burden. Hum Genomics. 2024;18(1):138. https://doi.org/10.1186/s40246-024-00700-x.

16. Aryayev M, Senkivska L, Lowe JB. Psycho-emotional and behavioral problems in children with growth hormone deficiency. Front Pediatr. 2021;9:707648. https://doi.org/10.3389/fped.2021.707648.

17. Fischer PR, Johnson CR, Leopold KN, Thacher TD. Treatment of vitamin D deficiency in children. Expert Rev Endocrinol Metab. 2023;18(6):489–502. https://doi.org/10.1080/17446651.2023.2270053.

18. Abuhamad AY, Almasri N, Al Karaghouli Y, Kadam R, Alhashmi M, Alzaabi E, Deeb A, Fischer PR. Vitamin D deficiency and associated demographic risk factors in children at a tertiary hospital in Abu Dhabi. Paediatr Int Child Health. 2024;44(3–4):105–10. https://doi.org/10.1080/20469047.2024.2396714.

19. Madkhali Y, Janakiraman B, Alsubaie F, Albalawi O, Alrashidy S, Alturki M, Ahmed M, Manzar MD, Kashoo F. Prevalence and trends of vitamin D deficiency in a Saudi Arabian population: a five-years retrospective study from 2017 to 2021. Front Public Health. 2025;13:1535980. https://doi.org/10.3389/fpubh.2025.1535980.

20. Hwalla N, Al Dhaheri AS, Radwan H, Alfawaz HA, Fouda MA, Al-Daghri NM, Zaghloul S, Blumberg JB. The prevalence of micronutrient deficiencies and inadequacies in the Middle East and approaches to interventions. Nutrients. 2017;9(3):229. https://doi.org/10.3390/nu9030229.

21. Hamali HA. An overview of the incidence, causes, and impact of iron deficiency anemia in Saudi Arabia. Clin Lab. 2025;71(4) https://doi.org/10.7754/Clin.Lab.2024.241102.

Chapter 5
Functional Disorders, Chronic Fatigue, Chronic Pain

Principles

Structural Disorders Are Common

We are fairly well trained to recognize structural disorders. When an adolescent presents with intermittent abdominal bloating and abdominal discomfort, we might find a normal physical exam but be prompted to check tissue transglutaminase IgA antibodies to diagnose celiac disease. If a patient presents with abdominal pain and intermittent bloody stools and has iron deficiency, we would suspect inflammatory bowel disease and consider endoscopic biopsies. If a patient has fatigue, we might notice an enlarged thyroid gland and an elevated thyroid stimulating hormone level. For a patient who has terrible headaches that wake the patient up during the night and are associated with vomiting, especially when we find papilledema on exam or see a mass on MRI review, we diagnose a brain tumor. These are examples of structural disorders for which a physical exam or testing (whether in a laboratory or via imaging or with biopsies or using other electrophysiologic exams such as an electrocardiogram or an electroencephalogram) helps lead us to diagnose a specific pathology of a specific organ or organ system.

Of course, acute conditions are often similarly identifiable by a physical exam and an abnormal test result, whether streptococcal pharyngitis or appendicitis or a forearm fracture. Overall, about 70% of medical visits are due to a specific, identifiable structural pathology.

A. J. Chattha et al., *Adolescent Medicine in the Middle East: Principles,
Perspectives, Practices,* https://doi.org/10.1007/978-3-032-12348-0_5

Functional Disorders Are Also Fairly Common

What about the other 30% of medical visits? How do we view the third of patients who present with bothersome symptoms not accompanied by any abnormal finding?

It is helpful to consider illnesses as either structural or functional. Structural disorders can be identified by physical exam and/or test abnormalities. Functional disorders result from brain-nerve dysfunction, causing symptoms without any specific pathology identified on evaluation of specific body parts.

Approximately 30% of medical visits are related to functional disorders. Examples of functional disorders include chronic migraine headaches, irritable bowel syndrome, and postural orthostatic tachycardia syndrome.

Functional Disorders—A Recent Study
A Middle Eastern cross-sectional school-based survey of 1200 adolescents (aged 12–18 years) identified functional gastrointestinal disorders in 27%. The risk was highest among girls, individuals with low physical activity, poor sleep, and a parental history of somatization. These data support incorporating functional disorder assessment into school health screening programs.

Vanitha A Jagannath, MBBS, MD
Manama, Bahrain

Words and Explanations Matter

Some physicians have the idea that structural disorders are real and function disorders are imaginary. Certainly, a patient with severe monthly headaches that are preceded by an aura, that are associated with vomiting, and that are relieved gradually by sleep, should not be told that a negative MRI study means the patient is normal. Rather, we would be able to diagnose a specific functional disorder, that of migraine headaches.

Gastroenterologists for many years have referred to "functional gastrointestinal disorders." We are shifting now to call these "disorders of gut-brain interaction." By whatever words, we should be careful that we are explaining situations without ever implying that a patient's concerns are unimportant or unreal. If a patient with abdominal problems has negative testing for both celiac disease and inflammatory bowel disease, that does not mean the patient is normal, even though some of the results are normal. Too many patients feel discounted when a physician looks at test results and concludes "you are normal."

Several Sorts of Functional disorders Are Fairly Well Characterized

Common to all functional disorders are the facts that these disorders are real, these disorders are bothersome and sometimes life-limiting, these disorders are associated with normal physical exams and testing, and these disorders follow identifiable patterns.

There are several forms of functional gastrointestinal disorders. Some patients have chronic nausea or dyspepsia. Others have dysmotility with irritable bowel syndrome. Others have constipation. These can be functional disorders without any identifiable exam or test result abnormality. The Rome Criteria provide diagnostic details (https://theromefoundation.org/rome-iv/rome-iv-criteria/, updated every few years).

There are several sorts of chronic pain syndrome. Specific headache patterns can be classified as migraines or cluster headaches or new chronic daily headaches. Pain limited to some body parts can be associated with specific features of chronic regional pain syndrome. Generalized systemic pain might fit diagnostic criteria for fibromyalgia. These pain syndromes are examples of functional disorders affecting the sensory nervous system.

Chronic fatigue, with or without the orthostatic intolerance and excessive postural tachycardia of postural orthostatic tachycardia syndrome, can be a functional disorder. Of course, some functional disorders can persist and are diagnosed after correcting other co-existing structural disorders such as hypothyroidism or iron deficiency.

In some situations, the dysfunctional body-brain connection seems to be more fully disrupted. Non-epileptic seizures and seeming blindness and paralysis (conversion) result when the brain's intended messages completely fail to be implemented by the body. Functional disorders can affect sensory, motor, and autonomic nervous systems. Functional disorders are distinct from but can interact with psychiatric disorders; functional disorders are not merely psychogenic.

The Underlying Goal of Adolescent Medicine Is to Develop **Appropriate** *Function*

Adolescent medicine is not like cosmetic surgery. Cosmetic surgeons seek to make patients look better. Clinicians caring for adolescents seek to help adolescents *become* adults, adults who *do well* and who *do good*, not just those who look good.

Thus, the care of adolescents aims to restore functional order, to help get the body and the person working well, cohesively. Clinicians should not simply focus on the eradication of disease or the removal of symptoms; rather, we should focus on what the adolescent becomes able to *do*. We work toward recovery from both structural and functional disorders to help the body's structures function well together.

Structural vs Functional Disorders—My Overview

Definition: Functional disorders are real disorders of brain-body communication without structural pathology.

Examples: migraine, irritable bowel syndrome, postural orthostatic tachycardia syndrome, chronic fatigue, conversion disorders

Key message: Normal tests do not mean absence of disease; they help define its nature.

Vanitha A Jagannath, MBBS, MD
Manama, Bahrain

Perspectives from the Middle East

As elsewhere in the world, patients and families in the Middle East have a variety of views of structural and functional disorders. Toward one extreme is the example of a boy with palpitations that the father attributed to excitement about girls; the boy had a cardiomyopathy with dysrhythmia. At another side of the spectrum was an adolescent with severe headaches. The father sought doctor after doctor requesting additional brain MRI studies; the father struggled to accept that headaches could come from something other than an anatomic abnormality in the brain and that surgery or medication wouldn't fix his child.

Similar to medical care in North America, clinicians in the Middle East are often required by their employers to see patients rapidly. Commercial interests prompt some health systems to prioritize testing over history-taking. As a result, many families expect that all diagnoses will come from tests and that chronic conditions for which test results have been normal simply require more or better testing.

Likewise, some medical training settings involve trainees starting care and then faculty members quizzing trainees about whatever tests they might have missed doing. Or, nurses might be empowered to initiate testing based on a chief complaint before a physician has even seen the child. While such practices might expedite the time course of diagnosing some structural problems, this style of care leaves patients and families thinking that all problems are structural or that functional problems are less important or less valid.

Practices in the Middle East

As we begin to take a history of an illness, we can ask how the symptoms alter function, subtly pointing at the value of *doing* something (functioning) instead of just being symptom-free. We can point to the journey through adolescence as we ask how the symptoms affect and perhaps alter plans to keep growing in certain areas. We show that we care about function and not just symptoms or structures.

We can then reflect with patients and families on what we are thinking, making comments about how a body part isn't working well even though it is not swollen or red or obviously diseased. We might suggest that even though a body part looks or tests as normal, there must be a problem in that body part's reception of messages from the brain since the body part is not doing what the person obviously wants it to do. Even with our reflective comments as we hear about the symptoms, we are preparing the patient for the possibility that the problem is functional rather than structural.

Part of getting the history of an illness, especially when the symptoms have recurred or persisted, is to ask what other doctors thought when they saw the patient. We ask not just what the diagnosis and treatment were, but we also ask how the clinician explained the symptoms, even after the test results were normal. In asking, we model openness to the possibility of alternate explanations for the symptoms. Then, we might tell the patient that we prefer to explain things differently, and then we do so in ways that do not diminish the validity of the patient's concerns.

Through all this, we accept the patient's report. We believe in the reality of the symptoms. (An exception would be when a patient has schizophrenia and does not accurately perceive reality. In that case, we respectfully propose an alternate view of reality.) Patients with chronic symptoms who feel like a physician is not validating the reality of the symptoms will then be unlikely to commit to following that physician's recommendations. Whether the disorder turns out to be structural or functional, we can validate the reality of the patient's symptoms. A wheelchair-bound adolescent was asked why she was quickly able to walk normally after seeing a specific clinician when she had only become more debilitated during months of seeing other doctors; "he believed me," she said. We can be careful not to discredit previous physicians, even if we express gratitude that the patient did well with the way we explained the situation.

Some clinicians tell patients that they will seek structural diagnoses and then consider a functional disorder (and helpful psychological therapy) if initial testing is normal. Patients often hear this as if they were told, "if we don't find anything wrong, the problem might be in your head and you'll need mental health help." It usually works better to pursue structural and functional diagnoses concurrently, especially since the two sometimes co-exist. Functional disorder diagnoses need not be diagnoses of exclusion and we can reach these diagnoses based on clear diagnostic criteria; at the same time, however, we might exclude contributing co-existing disorders and do tests to identify them.

We must be vigilant to avoid using words that suggest that normal results indicate that the patient is normal. We can say that the normal results show the absence of a specific problem with a particular body system, even as we continue to validate the reality of the symptoms.

> **Clear Communication—How I Do It**
> 1. Avoid stigma and build trust.
>   Examples:
>   *Your tests are normal, which is good news. They show your body parts aren't damaged. But your body isn't functioning well right now, and that's real. We can help retrain it.*
>
>   *Functional disorders are like having the wrong settings in your phone apps—everything is there, but it isn't working properly.*
> 2. Avoid implying that functional disorders are a "last resort" diagnosis.
>   Example:
>   *We will check for conditions affecting your stomach lining and also consider how your stomach nerves and brain signals are interacting.*
>
> Vanitha A Jagannath, MBBS, MD
> Manama, Bahrain

When we do want to get a psychologist involved, we need to explain that person's role carefully. We might say something like *I'd like you to see Dr X who has specific skills in helping patients with chronic pain.* We would then say that this person is a psychologist who is especially good at helping patients with good minds get their brains back in control of their bodies. Functional disorders are due to the brain and the body not communicating and coordinating actions well; these are not necessarily mental health disorders.

Whether we end up managing the patient for a structural or a functional disorder, or both, we can always work toward maximizing good function. We focus not just on the eradication of disease but, rather, on the restoration of normal function. We set treatment goals that relate to good function, such as making it to school on time, rather than on simply curing symptoms, such as morning vomiting.

For Reflection

Think about the last time a patient became frustrated when an evaluation for bothersome symptoms showed only normal results. How might you explain such findings next time?

Chronic Fatigue

Principles

Chronic Fatigue Is Common During Adolescence

About one-third of adolescents have bothersome fatigue that makes it difficult to get up and going at least twice a week. More than 20% of adolescent girls and approximately 7% of adolescent boys have had bothersome fatigue persisting more than three months. Between 1 and 2% of adolescents are disabled by fatigue and are unable to participate in routine daily activities. Fatigue is common!

Many Adolescents Have Chronic and/or Recurring Fatigue Due to Lifestyle Imbalances

Adolescents need about nine to nine and a half hours of sleep each night to maintain normally active lives. Unfortunately, the majority of adolescents get significantly less sleep than that. When an adolescent sleeps longer on a weekend when nothing is scheduled in the morning than on school days, the adolescent is suffering from a chronic sleep debt.

Lack of exercise also leaves adolescents feeling sluggish and tired. Irregular meal schedules also lead to tiredness. Much of the common adolescent chronic fatigue is due to lifestyle imbalances related to sleep, exercise, and meals.

Several Specific Medical Conditions Are Associated with Fatigue in Adolescents

Several organic (structural) medical conditions cause long-term fatigue in adolescents. Iron deficiency (with a ferritin level less than 20 ng/mL, with or without anemia) causes tiredness. Hypothyroidism causes tiredness, and Hashimoto thyroiditis is often at the base of adolescent hypothyroidism. Actual sleep disorders (beyond inadequate sleep duration) cause chronic fatigue; snoring would suggest obstructive sleep apnea, and leg pain with lots of tossing and turning during the night would suggest restless leg syndrome (periodic limb movement disorder). Celiac disease can cause fatigue, even without many gastrointestinal symptoms. Less commonly, renal insufficiency and autoimmune hepatitis can cause fatigue, even without other specific signs or symptoms of illness. The diagnosis and management of these conditions are relatively straightforward.

Chronic Fatigue Is Often Multifactorial

Most adolescents who struggle with chronic fatigue have several concurrent treatable conditions. They might be sleep-deprived and, separately, also have iron deficiency. They might have a structural (organic) cause of fatigue at the same time that they suffer from functional chronic fatigue.

Chronic Fatigue During Adolescence Is Often Linked to Autonomic Dysfunction

In adolescents, chronic fatigue is often associated with dizziness and/or gastrointestinal discomfort and/or irregular temperature sensations. These overlapping symptoms suggest that autonomic dysfunction might be at the foundation of the fatigue since it is the autonomic nervous system that normally regulates blood flow (without which altered blood flow to the body can lead to muscular fatigue and altered blood flow to the brain can lead to dizziness and mental clouding), gastrointestinal flow (without which there are functional gastrointestinal symptoms such as bloating, discomfort, and nausea), and temperature (which, when not well-regulated leads to feeling hotter or colder than peers in the same setting).

Autonomic dysfunction is a typical functional disorder and is sometimes even called an invisible disease since the person looks well with a normal physical exam and normal diagnostic test results. The problem is that the automatic or involuntary functions of the body are no longer adequately coordinated and controlled, and the dysfunctional autonomic system leads to fatigue and other symptoms. One specific form of autonomic dysfunction is postural orthostatic tachycardia syndrome (POTS). POTS is characterized by at least three months of orthostatic intolerance, usually with daily fatigue and often with abdominal symptoms, associated with an excessive (more than a 40 beat per minute change) increase in heart rate when going from supine resting to upright standing. Some studies suggest that most adolescents with chronic functional fatigue have some autonomic dysfunction, and a third or more have POTS.

Treatment of Chronic Fatigue Should Be Multifaceted

Each component of a patient's fatigue should be managed. Co-existing structural disorders should be treated. (About half of adolescents with POTS also have iron deficiency, and iron supplementation helps reduce the symptom burden.)

At the same time, the treatment of functional chronic fatigue also requires a team. The family and patient should join with the care team in ensuring good sleep quality and quantity, every night. The patient and family should commit to daily aerobic exercise, typically for at least half an hour; strength training can also be helpful. The care team needs to consistently stress the value of exercise since the fatigued patient usually lacks any motivation to exercise when feeling so tired. Having a personal trainer or coach or physical therapist can be helpful. The family and patient should work together to standardize schedules of healthy meals. Cognitive behavioral therapy is of proven effectiveness in overcoming chronic fatigue, so psychology input is useful.

Fatigued patients do best when they engage in regular school activities. Staying home and limiting activities serves only to worsen the fatigue. However, the school team should be supportive rather than punitive during the rare times that the patient is unable to either attend school or complete assignments in a timely fashion.

Chronic Fatigue Requires Chronic Treatment

Chronic fatigue is, well, chronic. It has lasted a long time. While there is good reason to stay optimistic about a full recovery, recovery can take months (or even years for some adolescents with POTS). The team must keep moving forward since good recovery with restoration of good activity is likely.

Words Matter

Some patients get consumed by internet information about "chronic fatigue syndrome" and end up either believing in unproven treatments or anticipating a lifelong condition. While "chronic fatigue syndrome" is a legitimate diagnosis for research studies, it is often more clinically useful to refer simply to "chronic fatigue" as validation that the tiredness has happened for a long time but with the anticipation that recovery is likely.

Perspectives from the Middle East

Teenagers are busy! In addition to schoolwork, many feel compelled by social pressure to engage in multiple extracurricular activities. Some move from one activity to the next and don't allow themselves enough down time to restore their minds and bodies. Over-activity, and the stress that commonly accompanies it, leads to tiredness.

In the Middle East, as in other parts of the well-resourced world, exercise is not often incorporated into regular adolescent routines. No longer do most teenagers walk to school or do vigorous physical chores around their homes. In some parts of the Middle East, daytime temperatures make outdoor activity very difficult during some parts of the year. Adolescents who do want to exercise might lack time or resources to get to an indoor gym. Whether from environmental situations, lack of motivation, or excessive time spent gaming and using electronic devices, exercise is not routine for most adolescents. The resulting lack of exercise, whether or not intentional, leads to worsened fatigue.

On the other hand, excessive exercise (without adequate intake to support it) is sometimes associated with restrictive energy intake disorder of sports (RED-S) and with anorexia. However, without these superimposed disorders, it is usually a *lack* of exercise that is more problematic in causing fatigue.

Surveys around the world (including those done in Middle Eastern countries) reveal that only a minority of adolescents get even the recommended minimum three hours of moderate to vigorous physical activity each week. This lack of exercise is associated with rising rates of obesity which provides yet another fatiguing factor. Lifestyle factors involving sedentary behaviors and weight gain are important in explaining an increasing frequency of chronic fatigue, and also in directing treatment for fatigue.

Reduced social contact, coupled with reduced exercise, during the COVID-19 pandemic sometimes led to emotional and then physical malaise. Without usual peer contacts, apathy and even depression ensued. Depression is usually accompanied by fatigue, and some adolescents found it difficult to return to normal activities post-pandemic due to ongoing fatigue.

Practices in the Middle East

Clinicians who are involved with adolescents can advocate for healthy lifestyles that will reduce fatigue in the population. They can also deal effectively with fatigue when it is identified.

For All Adolescents

As clinicians, we should encourage healthy lifestyles for all of our patients. In routine healthcare visits, we can advocate for adequate sleep, limited screen time, daily exercise, and balanced eating behaviors—all along with good social interactions.

Sleep. Adequate sleep is vital, and teenagers on average need nine or more hours each night of good quality sleep. Unfortunately, many adolescents in the Middle East are "so busy" with academic and extracurricular activities coupled with online "social" behaviors that they do not allow themselves enough time for restorative sleep. In fact, the average sleep duration for adolescents is between seven and eight hours per night. Clinicians should ask about sleep duration during healthcare visits and should point out how inadequate sleep compromises all aspects of health. Teens should be advised to avoid screen time during the hour before planned sleep and to allow for a good nine hours of sleep each night.

Device Use. Excessive screen time robs adolescents of time for more useful behaviors. There is no good reason for an adolescent to average more than two hours per day of non-educational (i.e., not for school work) screen time; this includes movies and videos and "web surfing" and social media use. Many adolescents in the Middle East spend six or more hours looking at their devices each day. Clinicians should encourage them to substitute screen time with behaviors that are more socially, educationally, and physically advantageous. Clinicians should remind their patients that there is no good reason for an adolescent to have more than two hours per day of non-educational screen time. Less screen time leads to more energy!

Eating. The adolescent body was designed to function with rhythms. Irregular eating schedules lead to tiredness and reduced productivity. Adolescents should be encouraged to eat regular meals each day, without skipping meals. Both irregular meal schedules and imbalanced dietary intake lead to fatigue.

Exercise. All adolescents should have at least three hours per week of moderate to vigorous physical activity. This can be integrated into normal, daily life routines. Clinicians can help their patients customize physical activity into their schedule, doing activities that adolescents enjoy.

Stress. Life is stressful, and we all use stress to motivate us toward good productivity. When stress interferes with relationships, sleep, and academic success, however, stress needs to be managed. Clinicians seeing adolescents should encourage them to balance busy times with calm times, to have confidants with whom they can speak, to identify role models who will help them process daily challenges, and, thus, to prevent energy-draining stress from leading to fatigue and poor outcomes.

For Tired Adolescents

Despite our best preventive efforts, however, we will continue to see tired adolescents. Sometimes, a history and physical exam will help identify a pathologic medical cause of the fatigue, but some structural disorders lack many specific symptoms and signs.

When an adolescent presents with persistent fatigue and there is no obvious singular cause on initial evaluation during a medical visit, laboratory testing is warranted.

Iron deficiency is common during adolescence, even in boys and even with seemingly normal diets. A low (<20 ng/mL) ferritin level indicates iron deficiency and should prompt treatment as well as a search for the cause (dietary insufficiency or malabsorption or blood loss) of the deficiency. A complete blood count could determine if there is also anemia (which can cause fatigue whether the anemia is due to iron deficiency or some other pathology). Ideally, the ferritin level would be checked when the patient is not ill with an inflammatory condition; otherwise, a C-reactive protein might help interpret the importance of the ferritin level, and testing iron binding saturation or a serum iron level can identify some iron-deficient patients. Iron deficiency itself is treated with 3–5 mg of elemental iron per kg of body weight per day, and dosing is best on an empty stomach and/or with vitamin C; related to the impact of hepcidin, daily dosing might be better than using divided doses. (Further details are in the chapter on Micronutrient Deficiencies.)

Hypothyroidism is common during adolescence, especially in females. An elevated thyroid stimulating hormone (TSH) level is usually adequate to identify hypothyroidism. If the level is elevated, checking for thyroperoxidase antibodies helps identify patients with Hashimoto thyroiditis. To identify the more rare patients with central hypothyroidism, adding a thyroxine (T4) level is helpful; checking free T4 is indicated since the free T4 is less likely altered by varying adolescent hormone levels.

Celiac disease can present with or without gastrointestinal symptoms in adolescents. Seeing a tired teen, testing a tissue transglutaminase antibody level should be considered.

Hidden renal and hepatic diseases less commonly cause fatigue. Nonetheless, it is reasonable to check renal function and a liver enzyme as screening tests in an adolescent with chronic fatigue.

Actual sleep disorders (beyond inadequate sleep) cause fatigue. A sleep study should be considered for tired adolescents who present with significant snoring, especially if they have daytime sleepiness (in addition to tiredness). Adolescents with unusual leg discomfort who move a lot during sleep hours might have restless leg syndrome (periodic limb movement disorder) which can be confirmed by overnight polysomnography and which can initially be treated with iron supplements to raise the ferritin level to above 50 ng/mL.

Adolescents presenting with chronic fatigue who also feel dizzy just after standing up might have autonomic dysfunction, whether or not their fatigue and dizziness are accompanied by abdominal symptoms or reported temperature dysregulation.

All patients with chronic fatigue and upright dizziness can benefit from increased fluid intake (enough so that the urine looks nearly water-like clear) and increased salt intake (as much added to their food as their tastebuds can tolerate). These patients should work up to 30 minutes of upright, daily, aerobic exercise. (The exercise is regimented and scheduled and should not depend on whether or not the patient feels like exercising.) Fatigue should *not* be a reason to limit academic activities. Cognitive behavioral therapy is of proven effectiveness for patients with chronic fatigue.

Patients presenting with findings suggestive of autonomic dysfunction should have a resting supine heart rate compared to the heart rate after three to five minutes standing up totally still. A supine-to-standing heart rate increase of more than 40 beats per minute is excessive postural tachycardia and suggests a diagnosis of postural orthostatic tachycardia syndrome. (In some centers, standardized tilt table testing is available for a more definitive diagnosis of POTS.) In addition to non-pharmacologic interventions for autonomic dysfunction, initial medication for POTS often includes metoprolol tartrate (25 mg by mouth first thing on awakening in the morning and again at mid-day) or midodrine (starting at 2.5 mg three times daily and increasing every five days if needed by 2.5 mg per dose up to a maximum of 10 mg three times daily; with attention for supine headaches which would limit the dose). Some experts also use fludrocortisone (0.1 mg by mouth once daily) though this is not usually necessary if the patient consumes adequate oral fluid and salt. Medications would be continued until a few months after the fatigue has resolved.

Recovery from functional chronic fatigue can take time. Compliance with treatment regimens is challenging for adolescents. It helps to have regular healthcare visits. Good communication between the patient, family, school, psychologist, and pediatrician can help ensure good outcomes.

For Reflection

A chronically tired adolescent refuses to accept your advice that exercise is an important step toward recovery, saying she just feels too tired. How will you respond?

Chronic Pain

Principles

Chronic Pain Is Common and Costly

Worldwide, according to various studies, 20–46% of adolescents suffer from chronic pain. Headache, abdominal discomfort, and musculoskeletal pain are typical forms of the pain that afflicts adolescents.

Adolescent pain compromises ease and effectiveness of daily activities. Pain impedes family and social interactions as well as academic progress. The adolescent years are vital in determining adult abilities and careers; loss of months of the adolescent years to pain results in limited adult potential. In the United States alone, healthcare costs for adolescent pain are 20 billion dollars or more per year.

Chronic Pain Often Follows a Structural Disorder But Persists After the Structural Condition Has Resolved

Acute injury and illness lead to inflammatory changes in tissues, altered neurochemistry in the dorsal horn, and changed neurotransmission in and between nerves, the spinal cord, and the brain. Likely related to the degree of initial biological changes but also to superimposed emotional and behavioral responses, pain can be propagated. Even after resolution of the initial inflammatory changes of peripheral tissues and central nervous system microglia, discomfort sometimes persists as chronic and/or recurring pain.

Of course, it is difficult to know just when acute pain (for which reductions in activity and responsibility can be appropriate treatment strategies) is transitioning to chronic pain (for which resumption of normal activities and responsibilities is essential). Sometimes, over-extending rest can lead to worsened long-term pain.

Chronic Pain Seems to Be Based in the Brain (Likely Hypothalamus) and Involves Altered Brain-Nerve-Organ Messaging

The shift from acute structural pain to chronic functional pain involves the resolution of peripheral inflammatory and neurochemical changes and the establishment of persistently altered neural pathways and, possibly, microglial inflammation. For at least some types of chronic pain, the hypothalamus is the site of altered microglia and nerve cell connectivity. An example is seen with allodynia when even light touch in specific anatomic areas of the body triggers a markedly exaggerated central sensation of extreme pain.

Altered mood can, thus, exacerbate chronic pain. Pain is depressing, but depression also has a detrimental effect on chronic pain. Serotonin-related neurotransmitters are likely involved in the central nervous system's regulation (and dysregulation) of chronic pain.

Understanding the Concept of "Central Sensitization" Can Be Helpful to Patients Dealing with Chronic Pain

In normal situations, the brain filters or limits the impact of incoming sensory input that serves minimal purpose. Thus, our brains do not continually register and "feel" the ongoing sensations of socks on ankles and collars on necks. Following initial episodes of discomfort (often extreme discomfort) in some predisposed adolescents, there is central sensitization whereby initially dysregulated peripheral and dorsal horn nerve function lead to persistently exaggerated (as if unfiltered) brain interpretation of pain. Some adolescents with chronic pain and central sensitization also report being consciously aware of the feelings of socks and collars and other normally ignored physical sensations.

Chronic Pain Can Be Managed with Multidisciplinary Care; Medications Serve an Adjunctive Role

Fortunately, good multidisciplinary care can lead to marked improvement in physical functioning despite pain and, eventually, resolution of the pain. Care team members can include family, school staff, physician(s), an experienced nurse-educator, and pain management psychologist(s). It is essential that participants in the recovery process provide consistent messages and input to guide recovery. Restoration of normal daily activities (regular meals, adequate sleep, daily exercise) and involvement of aggressive cognitive behavioral therapy strategies are critical to recovery. More than half of patients with chronic pain can benefit temporarily from the use of medication as they bridge toward recovery with non-pharmacologic strategies. While opioids can help with acute post-operative and post-injury pain, opioids are essentially never needed for adolescents with chronic pain; indeed, opioids can aggravate the disabilities caused by chronic pain.

Key Insights from the Middle East
Cultural and Social Context: Pain is often under-reported due to stigma, particularly among boys. Adolescents rely on family support, spirituality, and herbal remedies as coping strategies.

Healthcare Gaps: In Lebanon, 80% of healthcare professionals lack formal pediatric pain management education. Few specialized pediatric pain clinics exist across the region. Pain is often misdiagnosed or dismissed, delaying care and worsening outcomes.

Impact on Daily Life: Chronic pain contributes to school absenteeism, sleep disturbances, and emotional distress. Adolescents experience social withdrawal and a reduced quality of life.

Huda Abu-Saad Huijer RN, PhD, FEANS, FAAN
Balamand, Lebanon

Perspectives from the Middle East

Anecdotally, families in the Middle East have similarly varied responses to chronic pain as do families in other parts of the world. Some families confront chronic pain with a passion for more tests and a deeper search for a postulated quick cure. At the other end of the spectrum, some families settle in to accepting chronic pain as incurable and allow the child to become fully dependent on support systems while demanding stronger doses of chronic medicines while the adolescent becomes increasingly disabled. In between, some families come to grasp the reality of chronic pain as a functional disorder and are able to move toward a good recovery.

Cognitive behavioral therapy is an integral intervention in recovering from chronic pain. Usually, this is best managed by psychologists. However, good psychologists who have experience with cognitive behavioral therapy are not readily available in some parts of the Middle East. In fact, some psychologists might see a patient referred for chronic pain and decide "there is no psychological problem"—this can be completely true but is not helpful when the patient was referred for treatment of chronic pain rather than for an exploration of possible psychological problems. Clinicians might need to gain skills in cognitive behavioral therapy or identify helpful online resources to help patients in their particular settings.

At the same time, some patients, assuming that a referral to a psychologist implies that the pain is a "mental" problem or "all in my head," will decline a visit with a psychologist. Hopefully, a good discussion about the nature of functional disorders like chronic pain and a clear explanation of the desired role of the psychologist will help the patient gain enthusiasm for the possibility of cognitive behavioral therapy.

Challenges and Gaps
Lack of large-scale data on adolescent pain prevalence and risk factors.
Cultural barriers to acknowledging and treating pain.
Insufficient multidisciplinary services integrating physical, psychological, and family-based care.

Huda Abu-Saad Huijer RN, PhD, FEANS, FAAN
Balamand, Lebanon

Practices in the Middle East

Explore and Manage Contributing Factors

Many patients with chronic pain, as those with other functional disorders, have concurrent contributing conditions. It is important to manage each active medical issue.

From various research studies, 30–100% of patients with chronic pain have mild to moderate vitamin D deficiency. While severe vitamin D deficiency can cause uncomfortable bone and/or muscle disease, it is not clear whether mild and moderate hypovitaminosis D also play a causal role in adolescent chronic pain. It could be that adolescents with pain are less likely to spend time outdoors and then, secondarily, develop vitamin D deficiency. One way or the other, though, clinicians should ensure that adolescents with chronic pain have normal or normalizing vitamin D status.

Evidence of depression is found in 20–30% of adolescents with chronic pain. Sometimes depression pre-dates the onset of pain, and sometimes it seems that life changes caused by pain then subsequently lead to depression. However, since the same neurotransmitters implicated in the pathophysiology of depression are also involved in central pain pathways, it is likely that chronic pain and depression are concurrent downstream effects of underlying alterations in neurotransmitter function.

Hypermobility, as indicated by an elevated (>6) Beighton score, can lead to chronic joint pain. Physical therapists can help in strengthening muscles around the problematic joints and, thus, lead to reductions in pain intensity.

Extinguish Pain Behaviors

Acute pain prompts helpful behaviors to prevent aggravation of the pain. For instance, a broken leg hurts in ways that stop the patient from trying to bear weight, and ingestion of fatty foods by someone with gall bladder disease prompts pain that limits food intake. These are helpful behavioral responses to acute pain.

With chronic pain, however, altered nerve-behavior pathways end up exacerbating the pain. Abdominal wall muscle contraction makes chronic pain worse. Tightening neck muscles makes chronic headaches worse. Reductions in activity lead to increased levels of chronic pain. Even talking about chronic pain helps the body strengthen unhelpful nerve pathways and "nerve memory" and worsen the pain.

Thus, a foundation of an approach to chronic pain is to extinguish pain behaviors. Other than for rare medical monitoring of pain levels, the patient should not talk about the pain. The patient should not reduce regular activities. The patient should not grimace or double over or limp. Pain is reduced when pain behaviors are extinguished.

Patients with chronic abdominal or extremity pain might have altered their posture and gait. Physical therapists can help the patient eliminate their inadvertent postural and pain behaviors.

Extinguishing pain behaviors does not imply that the pain is not real. Rather, the reality of the pain is acknowledged even as pain management begins by eliminating all negative behavioral responses to the pain.

Parents who want to lovingly sympathize with a hurting child find it very difficult to extinguish pain behaviors, even to stop asking how the pain is. Parents as well as patients need to be informed of the value of "tough love" that eliminates pain behaviors as a means of eliminating the pain; this is the opposite of encouraging the pain by responding to it with unhelpful (and even harmful) behaviors.

Maximize Diet, Sleep, Exercise, and Regular School Activities

A normal response to pain is to decrease activity and to adapt schedules. This is effective for acute pain, but it is counter-productive for chronic pain.

Adolescents with chronic pain *must* be advised to normalize their eating and sleeping schedules. They should go to school regularly, even if it initially takes a few weeks of incremental schedule increases to achieve that goal.

Aerobic exercise facilitates recovery from chronic pain. Strengthening exercises helps uncomfortable extremities recover, and physical therapists can provide professional guidance for exercise programs. Stretching and massage can help soothe low back pain. Typically, the degree of chronic pain decreases as physical activity increases. Exercise should be planned and implemented according to that plan; other than delaying some exercise during moments of extreme headache, exercise plans should not be altered based on how the patient is feeling. (The pain is real but unhelpful. The patient's condition worsens with reductions in exercise. Exercise avoidance is a pain behavior to be extinguished.)

Explain Chronic Pain and Central Sensitization

Most adolescents are intelligent, especially when they have been reading about their chronic conditions. Unfortunately, not everything they read is helpful.

Clinicians caring for adolescents with chronic pain can provide good information, often with educational handouts and videos. Locally available internet sources can be reviewed for accuracy.

The pathophysiology of chronic pain, and how it differs from acute pain, should be discussed with patients. Adolescents often like "big words" and learning new concepts about pain processes. Many patients will not have heard about central sensitization and will grow to better understand their pain when they see it as neurologic filters that are stuck open and that are amenable to behavioral and thought changes that help close the filters. Testimonials from previous patients are available online and can help provide both information and peer encouragement.

Implement Cognitive Behavioral Therapy Strategies

Many pediatricians find that an experienced nurse educator and a psychologist with cognitive behavioral therapy skills are essential to their management of chronic pain. The *mood disorders* chapter of this book includes more details about some of the principles of cognitive behavioral therapy. Nurses, educators, and psychologists can help implement specific strategies with patients. Adjunct interventions involving distraction, relaxation, and mindfulness are also effective.

Consider Devices and Medications

Adolescents with localized chronic pain can benefit from use of a transcutaneous electrical nerve stimulation (TENS) unit. This device provides mild tingly sensations over a local body area. Nerves become accustomed to the sensation and stop noticing it (as if closing the filters of a person with central sensitization). The patient then subconsciously learns to stop noticing the pain whether the device is activated or not. This is particularly useful during the initial weeks of treating abdominal pain. Modifications of this device have been used intermittently on the forehead to reduce headaches.

Narcotics should always be avoided for adolescents with chronic pain. The risks (side effects such as sleepiness, constipation, and addiction) greatly outweigh the benefits (reduced pain intensity). In addition, narcotics dull mentation and make it harder for patients to stay active (when activity is a mainstay of therapy).

Some other medications, however, can help reduce (or even repair) altered pain nerve activity and can help patients implement the longer-term interventions (as reviewed above) that lead to improvement in daily function and to true recovery. Medication selection and dosing should be customized for each patient by a clinician with experience treating chronic pain in adolescents, but some guidelines follow.

Acute pain relief, especially for migraine headaches, can be provided by ibuprofen (10 mg/kg/dose, up to four times daily) and paracetamol (15 mg/kg/dose, up to six times daily). Using either of these medications more than three days in a week for chronic headaches, however, can lead to worsened rebound headaches. Triptans can also help for intermittent use in treating migraine headaches.

Amitriptyline (and its pharmacologic relative nortriptyline) were previously used for depression and seem to alter serotonin and norepinephrine uptake at nerve synapses; this can help some patients with chronic abdominal pain and/or frequent headaches. It is given daily by mouth, usually starting at about 0.5 mg/kg/dose and then increasing if needed to 1 or 2 mg/kg/dose. Propranolol (long-acting form, 1–2 mg/kg/dose given daily) can also help reduce headache frequency.

Citalopram increases synaptic activity of serotonin and can be useful for chronic or recurrent abdominal pain when given daily (10 mg initially, perhaps working up to 20 or even 40 mg per day). If there is concurrent depression, a psychiatrist can better help guide dosing. Duloxetine inhibits both serotonin and norepinephrine uptake in synapses and has been helpful for adults with fibromyalgia-like pains; fewer data are available supporting its use in adolescents.

Gabapentin is an oral anti-epileptic medication that also seems to moderate peripheral nerve conduction and to reduce neuropathic pain and headaches. Adolescents can start with 300 mg each evening and add/increase a dose every three days as needed; some require up to 1200 mg three times daily. This medication, like citalopram and duloxetine, should not be stopped abruptly but should be weaned gradually, reversing the dosing changes used at initiation. Gabapentin is also effective for patients with restless leg syndrome who do not adequately respond to aggressive iron supplementation.

Other medications, some related to the ones mentioned here, can also be used for chronic pain in adolescents. However, these medications all act on the nervous system and should be used with appropriate caution by clinicians who have experience in using them.

> **Recommendations**
> Conduct national and regional studies to quantify prevalence and identify risk factors.
> Train healthcare professionals in pediatric pain assessment and management.
> Establish multidisciplinary pain centers tailored for adolescents. Involve clinical nurse specialists specialized in pain management
> Incorporate culturally sensitive strategies, including family engagement and community education.
> Raise awareness in schools and communities to reduce stigma and encourage early reporting.
>
> Huda Abu-Saad Huijer RN, PhD, FEANS, FAAN
> Balamand, Lebanon

For Reflection

A parent insists that you provide a prescription for a narcotic for an adolescent with chronic pain. How can you stay therapeutically aligned with the patient and family while believing that such a prescription would actually decrease the potential for recovery?

Further Reading

1. Sunde KE, Hilliker DR, Fischer PR. Understanding and managing adolescents with conversion and functional disorders. Pediatr Rev. 2020;41(12):630–41. https://doi.org/10.1542/pir.2019-0042.
2. Kizilbash SJ, Ahrens SP, Bruce BK, Chelimsky G, Driscoll SW, Harbeck-Weber C, Lloyd RM, Mack KJ, Nelson DE, Ninis N, Pianosi PT, Stewart JM, Weiss KE, Fischer PR. Adolescent fatigue, POTS, and recovery: a guide for clinicians. Curr Probl Pediatr Adolesc Health Care. 2014;44(5):108–33. https://doi.org/10.1016/j.cppeds.2013.12.014.
3. Stewart JM, Boris JR, Chelimsky G, Fischer PR, Fortunato JE, Grubb BP, Heyer GL, Jarjour IT, Medow MS, Numan MT, Pianosi PT, Singer W, Tarbell S, Chelimsky TC. Pediatric writing group of the American autonomic society. Pediatric disorders of orthostatic intolerance. Pediatrics. 2018;141(1):e20171673. https://doi.org/10.1542/peds.2017-1673.
4. Fischer PR. Tired teens. Mayo Clinic Press; 2021.
5. Landry BW, Fischer PR, Driscoll SW, Koch KM, Harbeck-Weber C, Mack KJ, Wilder RT, Bauer BA, Brandenburg JE. Managing chronic pain in children and adolescents: a clinical review. PMR. 2015 Nov;7(11 Suppl):S295–315. https://doi.org/10.1016/j.pmrj.2015.09.006.

Chapter 6
Managing: Chronic Structural Disorders

Principles

Set Realistic Expectations

The overarching theme in managing chronic diseases in the Middle East is regular, realistic conversations with patients and their families about expectations. A complete cure is usually impossible, yet most patients can live and function much closer to their ideal than they realize. Focus on small, achievable steps and regular follow-up.

Prioritize a Primary-Care Relationship with the Patient

In line with this, choose to become a primary care physician, regardless of your specialty, in the sense that you prioritize and value caring for a patient over the long term. Emphasize and encourage regular follow-up, even though families may not be familiar with this concept and it may not be an accepted part of the local health system. Prioritize preventative counseling, as you may be one of the only people to whom adolescents will listen. Experiment with various payment models in your private clinic that make regular follow-up affordable for families.

A. J. Chattha et al., *Adolescent Medicine in the Middle East: Principles, Perspectives, Practices*, https://doi.org/10.1007/978-3-032-12348-0_6

Be Mindful of the Whole Family

Engage the whole family every time you see them. These patients are an integral part of a wider circle of relatives, and their identities to some degree are wrapped up in the identities of their caregivers, and vice versa.

Be Mindful of What Is Available and How Much It Costs

This does not apply to all practice settings in the Middle East, but you may need to get comfortable prescribing what many in the West would call second line therapies. Glucocorticoids will often have to be substituted for biologics, NPH insulin may have to suffice in the place of glargine, and topical therapies for acne will likely be more affordable than oral retinoids.

Learn to Be a Physical Therapist (Sort of)

Physical therapy is a huge need for adolescents with motor dysfunction, yet there are not nearly enough physical therapists, and their services are often expensive, especially given that multiple sessions or even lifelong interventions will be needed. Physicians would do well to take courses or educate themselves about basic physical therapy techniques that can be taught and demonstrated during follow-up visits with patients. Organizations such as the International Committee of the Red Cross, Physiopedia, and Hambisela offer helpful courses in this regard.

Connect Your Patients with Each Other

Though types of chronic diseases vary widely, adolescents with chronic diseases often have a lot in common with each other. Though the symptoms are different, the experience of being a "chronically ill" adolescent can be remarkably similar. Seeking to bring together these patients in healthy support groups or to simply introduce the parents and families to each other can have a great impact on the patient's quality of life. There's growing evidence that patients do not all have to have the same chronic disease to support each other.

Watch for Risky Behaviors and Check on Mental Health Regularly

It is important to remember that adolescents with chronic diseases are still adolescents. Risky behaviors, such as tobacco use, occur at the same rate in these patients as they do in adolescents without chronic disease. Unfortunately, these behaviors may exacerbate their underlying chronic illness or interfere with appropriate treatment. Coupled with the fact that these adolescents have a higher rate of psychological comorbidities, it is essential that health care providers intentionally ask about and maintain awareness of the patient's social and psychological health.

Help the Patient Grow into an Adult Who Manages His/Her Own Chronic Disease

This unique stage of life is a crucial time for the patient to grow in self-management of their chronic illness. On the physician's part, a combination of teaching, encouraging self-monitoring, regular review of practice (along with troubleshooting) and a written action plan has been shown to help these adolescents make this crucial transition to adulthood.

Perspectives from the Middle East

Prevalence of chronic disease in the middle east

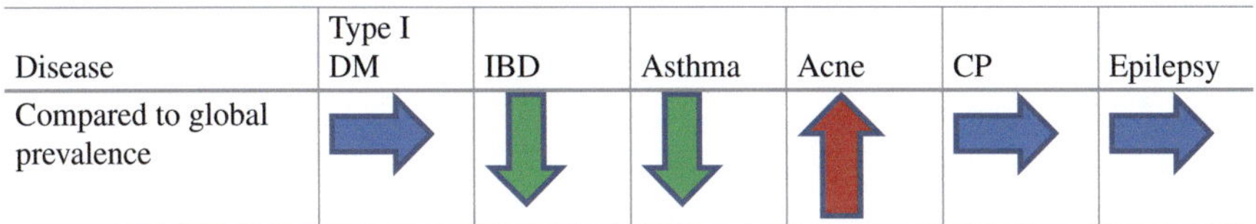

Disease	Type I DM	IBD	Asthma	Acne	CP	Epilepsy
Compared to global prevalence	→	↓	↓	↑	→	→

DM = Diabetes Mellitus; IBD = Inflammatory Bowel Disease; CP = Cerebral Palsy

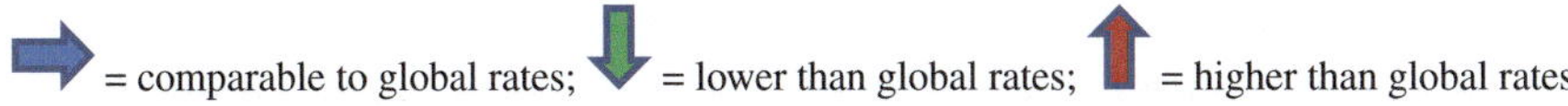

= comparable to global rates; = lower than global rates; = higher than global rates

While we want to be careful about generalizations, the cultural and social fabric of the Middle East is much tighter knit than that of the Western world, meaning that more value is placed on extended family relationships and especially on the authority that parents carry over their children. The physician will need to be aware of the autonomy (or lack thereof) that the patient has within their relationship with their parents. Physicians should engage the patient and parents actively, both together and individually, to see the best possible health outcomes.

Physicians should bear in mind the higher rate of illiteracy in the Middle East, especially among women. As professionals who are highly educated and perhaps take their literacy for granted, we should be careful to explain and teach at an appropriate level and be quick to reject any arrogance in our own attitudes.

The Muslim faith is widespread within the Middle East, and many patients and families will be devoted to this way of life. One tenant of Islam is accepting difficulty and illness from God with trust that He is all-powerful and sovereign. In the setting of a child with chronic disease, this attitude is often very visible in parents and will inform the treatments they choose and pursue. "If God wills" is an oft-spoken phrase. At the same time, as is the case all over the world, parents are often expecting or hoping for a definitive, preferably quick, cure for their child. This tension of what could be called 'fatalism' and expectation of a cure is a difficult one to maintain for physicians, as they encourage active treatment while acknowledging the long-term nature of the illness.

Though this varies by country, in general, Middle Eastern healthcare systems are not set up with multidisciplinary teams. The public/private system dynamic in many countries incentivizes individual physicians to remain independent of other healthcare providers. This complicates the management of adolescents with chronic diseases, often leading to fragmented care without a single primary care provider helping to keep the big picture.

Cost and availability of medications is a big determinant of the treatment plan for adolescents with chronic disease. Availability of medications, especially first-line therapies, is shifting constantly, and these drugs are often expensive. A lower daily wage means that even marked-down second-line therapies may be difficult for families to afford.

Practices in the Middle East

Type I Diabetes

Realistic goals for the patient and family are important. Without access to advanced insulin delivery technology or continuous glucose monitoring, a HgbA1c goal of <7.5 is reasonable, and a goal of <8 can be considered in situations where patient's life expectancy is limited or has a history of severe hypoglycemia. If HgbA1c testing is too expensive, control can be monitored through frequent morning fasting glucose checks.

Given the tight knit nature of families, it is imperative to include the whole family in the administration and management of insulin. Parents should be observed administering insulin, and the physician should troubleshoot and discuss the plan with the whole family.

Insulin therapy for these patients generally falls into two phases: the initial optimization phase and the long-term management phase. Both of these phases require frequent visits. While basal-bolus insulin regimens are ideal, cost and availability issues may force physicians to consider pre-mixed insulin alternatives. Worsening of glycemic control in adolescence is common. The onset of puberty brings physiologic changes that affect blood glucose. Increasing conflict with parents can lead to either limited or excessive involvement of the parents, both of which can have negative effects on glycemic control.

Be on the lookout for other adolescent issues that will interact significantly with diabetes. Diabetes distress includes fear of hyper/hypoglycemia, anxiety, depression, and disordered eating behaviors. A general increase in risky behavior will also pose more of a danger to the adolescent with a condition that requires frequent checks and intervention.

Inflammatory Bowel Disease

Peak onset of IBD is during adolescence, and incidence rises as countries become more developed. The two types are Crohn's disease (CD) and ulcerative colitis (UC), with CD being more common. CD can involve any part of the gastrointestinal tract, while UC is limited to the colon and sometimes the terminal ileum (backwash ileitis). CD also tends to have more perianal involvement. In UC, the Pediatric UC Activity Index (PUCAI) is used to assess severity of disease and guide treatment.

The general goal is to see mucosal healing. However, this requires treatment with biologics and regular endoscopy, both of which may be cost-prohibitive or unavailable. Glucocorticoids are an imperfect option, due to adverse effects. But they are likely the most affordable option to achieve remission. Exclusive enteral nutrition (EEN) can also achieve remission but is significantly more resource intensive. Aminosalicylates (mesalamine, balsalazide) can be used for maintenance of remission but are more effective for UC rather than CD. Immunomodulators such as thioprines and methotrexate have good success in maintenance of remission, especially for those whose disease is refractory to aminosalicylates. Anti-tumor necrosing factor (anti-TNF) biologics have revolutionized the treatment of IBD and should be used when possible. Surgery is also sometimes needed for refractory complications (including fistulas and strictures).

Adolescents should be monitored closely for micronutrient deficiencies and issues with growth and bone health. Most patients will need vitamin D supplementation. Cancer surveillance with endoscopy is indicated every one to two years. As in other chronic diseases, psychosocial symptoms, depression, and anxiety are all more common for patients with IBD.

Asthma

Asthma is usually diagnosed in childhood and early adolescence. Peak expiratory flow (PEF) is a cheaper alternative to spirometry for diagnosis.

Per the Global Initiative for Asthma (GINA) guidelines, there are two tracks for management of asthma, each involving a stepwise approach to escalating therapy, based on patient's symptom control. The preferred track is the use of an inhaled corticosteroid (ICS)/ long-acting beta-agonist (LABA) combination for both intermittent relief and maintenance therapy. The use of this combination inhaler begins from the time of the patient's diagnosis, where it is used as an intermittent "rescue" inhaler. These combination inhalers are available in the Middle East but are generally more expensive than the medications used in the second track.

The second track is the more traditional approach to asthma treatment, starting with a short-acting beta agonist (SABA) inhaler for intermittent treatment. GINA now recommends that an ICS inhaler be used in combination with a SABA, beginning from the first step of this track. Both tracks escalate treatment by first scheduling the use of the ICS or ICS/LABA inhaler, then increasing dosing of this maintenance therapy.

Acne

Research from the Middle East shows that acne generally worsens in the summer. Patients often perceive it as a cosmetic problem and therefore seek advice from beauticians rather than physicians. There is evidence to suggest an association between acne and a Western diet, which is something to be aware of as Western influences increase across the Middle East.

Middle Eastern adolescents more commonly have darker skin phototypes, which increases their risk of post inflammatory hyperpigmentation (PIH), a sequela of acne. Retinoids combined with benzoyl peroxide or salicylic acid have shown good results in reducing PIH.

The initial step in approaching acne is the assessment of lesions and classification of severity. The extent of skin involvement, presence/absence of nodules, associated scarring, and prominence of papules/pustules are criteria used to classify severity.

Managing Mild-Moderate Acne

MILD		MODERATE	
Comedonal	Papular/pustular	Papular/pustular	Moderately Severe
Topical Retinoid > Azelaic Acid > Salicylic Acid	Fixed Combination or BPO or Topical Retinoid or Azelaic Acid	Fixed Combination Preferred	Fixed Combination + Oral Antibiotic Preferred Or + Oral isotretinoid Or + Oral Zinc* Or + Oral Hormonal Therapy

If patient responds, treat until clear or almost clear

Maintenance Therapy:*	Topical Retinoid or Retinoid/BPO Combination

Actions if Response is Poor

✓ Check non-drug related reasons (seborrhea, stress and diet, malassezia furfur, G-bacteria, comedogenic skin care products, endocrine profile)
✓ Check drug-related reasons (adapt vehicle to skin type and environmental conditions, change topical agent, mechanically remove comedones, change from monotherapy to fixed-combination, change to higher concentration of topial). For females, check type of contraception.
✓ Probe patient's adherence (application technique, missed doses, tolerability)
✓ Ask about adverse events

From Gollnick H, Abanmi AA, Al-Enezi M, et al. Managing acne in the Middle East: consensus recommendations. *Journal of the European Academy of Dermatology and Venereology*. 2017;31:4–35. doi:10.1111/jdv.14491 used with permission

Parents and the patient need to be counseled on the time it takes to see improvement, the need for treatment adjustments along the way, and the need for maintenance. Skin hygiene should be reviewed.

Mild acne is usually treated with topical retinoids, topical antibiotics, and/or benzoyl peroxide. Adapalene 0.1% / benzoyl peroxide 2.5% is one commonly available combination topical treatment in the Middle East. It is generally not recommended to use oral or topical antibiotics as monotherapy. Moderate to severe acne is treated with oral isotretinoin if possible. Alternatives are oral antibiotics, oral contraceptives (for females), and spironolactone, all used in combination with topical therapies. Topical retinoids are the preferred maintenance therapy.

Neuromuscular Disorders

Epilepsy

The most commonly reported risk factor in the Middle East for epilepsy is parental consanguinity. Perinatal infections/insults and family history of epilepsy are also significant risk factors.

In an adolescent who has had their first unprovoked seizure, antiepileptic drugs are generally not indicated. Unprovoked means that the seizure is not in response to an acute infection, toxic or metabolic disturbance, head trauma or stroke.

The risk of second seizure should be evaluated, however, and antiepileptics discussed if appropriate. Risk factors for recurrent seizures include family history of epilepsy, abnormal EEG or MRI, focal seizure and/or prior neurologic insult. If a second unprovoked seizure occurs, antiepileptic should be started, based on the type of seizure. Levetiracetam is a common choice, given its broad-spectrum activity and minimal drug interactions. It is widely available in the Middle East.

Adherence to daily medication is challenging for adolescents. As with other chronic diseases, great care must be given to cultivating a trusting relationship with the patient and the family. Regular follow-up can help establish this therapeutic relationship. After 18 to 24 months without seizures, the physician can consider withdrawing antiepileptic medication. These drugs should be tapered.

Cerebral Palsy

This condition encompasses a wide range of permanent motor dysfunction resulting from in-utero or peri-birth insults to the brain. The risk of developing CP is increased by consanguinity, something that is more common in the Middle East.

By definition, these dysfunctions are not progressive, but their manifestation may change as the child grows and reaches adolescence. The most common type reported in the Middle East is spastic quadriplegia. Assessing and monitoring function over time is essential, using standardized measures such as the Gross Motor Function Classification System (GMFCS). Approximately half of children with CP in the Middle East are GMFCS IV or V (most severe classification is V). This is high relative to high-income countries.

The management of CP is ideally highly multidisciplinary with particular attention paid to altered motor tone and function. Physical therapy is the mainstay of treatment, while anti-spasticity drugs (baclofen being the most widely available) can be helpful adjuncts. Orthopedic assessment is helpful, but care should be taken in selecting invasive interventions such as musculoskeletal surgery or casting. Many have poor evidence of benefit, especially if used without intensive physical therapy follow-up. By the time a child with cerebral palsy reaches adolescence, they and their parents have likely settled into some type of routine and approach to daily living with their unique limitations. These routines can be healthy or unhealthy to varying degrees. It's important to review and explore all of these routines as a physician. Given the chronicity of the disease and intensive caregiving required, emotional and social support is key, and often the most helpful thing a physician can offer is a listening ear.

Evaluation and long-term management of various associated conditions is also key. These conditions include sleep disturbance, intellectual disability, nutrition, constipation, and communication, to name a few. The physician should work through these sequelae methodically and especially seek to optimize nutrition, sleep, and bowel function.

For Reflection
What are ways that you can adapt your practice to offer longitudinal primary care to adolescents with chronic diseases?

Further Reading

1. Sawyer SM, Drew S, Yeo MS, Britto MT. Adolescents with a chronic condition: challenges living, Challenges Treating. Lancet. 2007;369(9571):1481–9. https://doi.org/10.1016/S0140-6736(07)60370-5.
2. American Diabetes Association Professional Practice Committee. Children and adolescents: standards of medical Care in Diabetes-2022. Diabetes Care. 2022;45(Suppl 1):S208–31. https://doi.org/10.2337/dc22-S014.
3. Rosen MJ, Dhawan A, Saeed SA. Inflammatory bowel disease in children and adolescents. JAMA Pediatr. 2015;169(11):1053–60. https://doi.org/10.1001/jamapediatrics.2015.1982.
4. Mitchel EB, Rosh JR. Pediatric Management of Crohn's disease. Gastroenterol Clin N Am. 2022;51(2):401–24. https://doi.org/10.1016/J.GTC.2021.12.013.
5. Global Initiative for Asthma – GINA. 2024 GINA Main Report. https://ginasthma.org/2024-report.
6. Gollnick H, Abanmi AA, Al-Enezi M, Al Hammadi A, GaLADARI I, Kibbi AG, Zimmo S. Managing acne in the Middle East: consensus recommendations. J Eur Acad Dermatol Venereol. 2017;31:4–35. https://doi.org/10.1111/jdv.14491.
7. Mushta SM, King C, Goldsmith S, Smithers-Sheedy H, Badahdah AM, Rashid H, Badawi N, Khandaker G, McIntyre S. Epidemiology of cerebral palsy among children and adolescents in Arabic-speaking countries: a systematic review and meta-analysis. Brain Sci. 2022;12(7):859. https://doi.org/10.3390/brainsci12070859.
8. Idris A, Alabdaljabar MS, Almiro A, Alsuraimi A, Dawalibi A, Abduljawad S, AlKhateeb M. Prevalence, incidence, and risk factors of epilepsy in Arab countries: a systematic review. Seizure. 2021 Nov;92:40–50. https://doi.org/10.1016/j.seizure.2021.07.031.

Chapter 7
Mood Disorders

We mentioned that there are two types of health problems. First, structural disorders occur when the brain functions normally but a specific bodily organ/structure is diseased and not working well. Second, functional disorders occur when both the brain and the body seem individually normal but the brain and body are not communicating, connecting, and coordinating normally. In fact, there is also a third sort of disorder, psychiatric disorders.

Some people like to use a computer analogy to describe the various sorts of medical problems. When a computer is not working, the problem could be structural with damaged hardware. Alternatively, the problem could be "functional" with corrupted software. Finally, the problem could be psychiatric in origin with an altered central processing unit.

In psychiatric disorders, the brain, or mind, has altered thought processes and is not functioning normally. While there can be physical, structural correlates to psychiatric disorders (such as tachycardia with anxiety), the fundamental abnormality with psychiatric disorders is that of altered thinking. In some serious psychiatric disorders, thought processes are deeply affected, with major alterations in perceptions of reality as seen in psychoses. The altered thinking can, in other situations, be relatively mild as seen in patients with mood disorders, as discussed in this chapter, who have thoughts of "everything is bad, hopeless" with depression or thoughts and feelings of "things will never work out" with anxiety.

© The Author(s), under exclusive license to Springer Nature
Switzerland AG 2025
A. J. Chattha et al., *Adolescent Medicine in the Middle East: Principles,
Perspectives, Practices*, https://doi.org/10.1007/978-3-032-12348-0_7

Principles

Mood Changes Are Common, Multi-factorial, and Expected During Adolescence

The adolescent years can be tumultuous. Perspectives change as adolescents begin to see underlying issues and to seek deeper meaning in life. Peer groups can provide encouragement, yet also stress. Social media prompts some teens to adopt unrealistic expectations. And, as puberty progresses, adolescents can become increasingly self-conscious and, perhaps, hyper-critical of self. Emotions rise and fall. Moodiness shifts with hormonal changes and with varying life situations and experiences.

Thus, it is normal for moods to rise and fall during the adolescent years. Mood swings are to be expected. At the same time, though, adolescents can still be held accountable for their behavior. Mood changes can be uncomfortable for the adolescent and for everyone around the adolescent; mood changes feel bad! But, bad behavior is neither normal nor acceptable.

Mood Disorders Are More Extreme Situations that Alter Daily Success and Productivity

Sometimes, however, changes in mood become more extreme. Whether due to heightened anxiety or depressed moods, daily life becomes more challenging, relationships are strained, and academic performance suffers. When altered moods go beyond discomfort to dysfunctional, it is possible that there is an actual mood disorder.

Anxiety (generalized anxiety disorder) and depression are common adolescent mood disorders. More than a fourth of adolescents are affected by these disorders, either acutely or chronically.

While worry and nervousness are normal aspects of the adolescent years, an actual anxiety disorder is characterized by the frequency (multiple days each week, often with pervasive thoughts out of proportion to the external stressors) and severity (often with bodily symptoms, usually impairing daily function) of the worry and nervousness. Approximately 25% of adolescents experience anxiety, but only a minority of these patients are actually diagnosed with and treated for anxiety. In adolescents, anxiety often is present concurrently with attention deficit hyperactivity disorder, autism spectrum disorder, and depression.

In 2015, it was reported that 18% of girls and 8% of boys had experienced major depressive disorder by the end of the adolescent years; depression has become even more common since then, partly related to challenges prompted by the COVID-19 pandemic. Nearly a third of teens with depression will sometimes feel suicidal, and about 10% make an attempt to end their lives. Having a first-degree relative with depression is a significant risk factor for depression, as are adverse childhood experiences. Societal factors, including those related to social media overuse and addiction, also contribute to depression. Globally, depression is thought to account for more adult disability than any other condition. Suicide is one of the most common causes of death among North American adolescents.

Depression can persist chronically. In addition, major depressive episodes can occur with or without chronic depression. Major depression episodes persist for up to two months, and recurrence is common (about 30% within two years and about 70% within five years).

The Prevalence of Depression and Anxiety During Adolescence Is Increasing

During the past two decades, anxiety and depression and self-harm have become much more common during adolescence. In girls, prevalences have doubled; in boys, the prevalence of mental health disorders has gone up by about 40%.

Societal Factors Are Linked to the Increase in Mental Health Disorders During Recent Decades

Social psychologists have identified two disturbing trends that are causally associated with increasing mental health disorders during adolescents. Then, social isolation during the COVID-19 pandemic made the situation even worse.

First, in many resource-rich countries, concerns for child safety prompted parents to restrict independent and peer play by their children. Unstructured neighborhood play became less common. This prompted children to miss out on routine, daily unstructured interactions with peers that, for previous generations, had provided opportunity to learn to discern social cues, to develop self-governing safety practices, and to gain inter-personal relational skills. Less unstructured play during childhood is associated with more anxiety and depression during adolescence.

Second, the advent of continuous access to social media around 2015, while providing some educational information, resulted in girls, especially, being subjected to increasing pressures to look and behave in near-perfect fashion. Boys, at the same time, engaged increasingly in impersonal "games" of violence and domination. Using social media without in-person interactions left adolescents increasingly unprepared to foster healthy adolescent identity development and a realistic sense of importance.

Thus, reductions in unstructured play for children and increases in artificialized peer pressure through social media have altered pediatric development and contributed to increased prevalences of mental health disorders. The percents of adolescents affected by anxiety, depression, and eating disorders have skyrocketed.

Screening Helps Identify Adolescents Who Might Have an Actual Mood Disorder

Some clinicians use simple screening surveys to identify patients who might have an actual mood disorder worthy of specific treatment. Patients can either be screened at all visits or with check-ups and chronic care visits. It is important, though, that screening clinicians be able and available to promptly review results of the screening survey and to quickly and appropriately deal with abnormal findings.

Several screening tools are available to identify adolescents who might have significant anxiety. The seven-question generalized anxiety disorder (GAD-7) assessment has been validated with adolescents and is commonly used. Adolescents only need one to two minutes to rate the frequency of the symptoms noted in the survey's seven questions. The screening tool and scoring system are available online (https://adaa.org/sites/default/files/GAD-7_Anxiety-updated_0.pdf) in English, Arabic, and a few other languages (https://www.phqscreeners.com/select-screener).

The nine-question patient health questionnaire (PHQ-9) is useful in identifying adolescents at risk of having significant depression. It, too, is validated, readily available online (https://med.stanford.edu/fastlab/research/imapp/msrs/_jcr_content/main/accordion/accordion_content3/download_256324296/file.res/PHQ9%20 id%20date%2008.03.pdf), and easy to complete quickly. It is recommended that each adolescent complete the depression screen at least annually. Adolescents with risk factors for depression (positive family history of depression or bipolar disorder or suicide or substance abuse) might benefit from more frequent screening. A high score or positive screening test does not necessarily prove a diagnosis of depression but should prompt a one-on-one clinical evaluation as well as a confidential discussion with a parent. During that evaluation, depression, as distinct from mere sadness, would be associated with functional impairment of self-care, academic performance, social engagement, and/or completion of assigned responsibilities (such as chores at home).

Anxiety and Depression Are Treatable

Even in North America with an advanced workforce of child psychiatrists, approximately half of adolescents with depression are not appropriately diagnosed. The majority of care is provided by primary care providers. However, with good, routine screening, the diagnosis can be readily made. Good guidelines exist to guide therapy and pharmacologic management.

Symptoms and Signs of More Extreme Psychological Imbalance Should Prompt Referral for Specialty Care

An initial evaluation of an adolescent with a possible mood disorder can often be accomplished by a pediatrician or primary care clinician. Concurrently contributing comorbid medical conditions, such as hypothyroidism and anemia and eating disorders, can be ruled out or treated. Suggested therapies may be initiated, as might be initial medications. However, comprehensive management of moderate to severe anxiety and depression can be best facilitated by a psychiatrist who is experienced with medication management.

It is also common to involve a psychiatrist in medication management when an adolescent with depression also has episodes of hypomania or mania (with excessive energy, reduced sleep, rapid speech, and distractibility). Bipolar disease is possible in such patients, and medication choices differ from those of children with less complicated depression.

Various Forms of Therapy Can Be Useful, Even from Within a Pediatric Practice

As described below, cognitive behavioral therapy can be effectively initiated by pediatricians and primary care providers, especially when psychologists who have experience with cognitive behavioral therapy are not available. Similarly, acceptance and commitment therapy can also be useful for many adolescents.

Medications Are Sometimes Necessary and Helpful. Psychiatry Colleagues Should Be Consulted Appropriately

When symptoms are severe and/or when symptoms persist despite initial efforts at non-pharmacologic treatment, medications may be indicated. Selective serotonin reuptake inhibitors are usually safe and are often effective in adolescents. When available, psychiatrists can assist with medication dosing and management.

Perspectives from the Middle East

A 2022 study published in the *British Journal of Clinical Psychology* evaluated the global prevalence of depressive symptoms in adolescents. The highest prevalences were noted in the Middle East, Africa, and Asia; rates had increased during the previous two decades. Depression is clearly a major issue among adolescents in the Middle East. As elsewhere, rates of adolescent mood disorders in the Middle East climbed during the COVID-19 pandemic.

Several Middle Eastern nations have suffered from wars and conflict during recent years. Families have been displaced within or beyond their home countries. Lives have been lost. These tragic situations have led to increased incidences of anxiety and depression in addition to other mood disorders and post-traumatic stress disorder. Anxiety disorders related to civil unrest were already common in Palestine prior to the 2023–2024 escalation in conflict.

In wealthier areas of the Middle East, alterations in childhood play and adolescent exposure to social media have increased the risk of mental health disorders in ways paralleling the situation in wealthy North American and European countries. Seasonal weather patterns alter some unstructured outdoor play, and the availability of engagement with private, indoor social media further deprives adolescents of healthy in-person contact that is necessary for healthy adolescent development.

In the Middle East, as in other regions of the world, there are varied reactions to mood disorders. Sometimes, the problem is minimized with simple suggestions such as "relax, sleep better, don't worry, think positively." These actions can be helpful, especially for adolescents merely going through mood changes, but these suggestions are clearly inadequate for patients with actual mood disorders. Other times, mood disorders are stigmatized, and affected adolescents are seen as weak and their struggles as insignificant; again, these reactions are unhelpful, wherever in the world they occur.

Adolescents in many regions within the Middle East lack optimal access to mental health professionals. Skilled psychologists and psychiatrists with adolescent expertise are not always readily available. This leaves primary care providers shouldering a large part of the burden of adolescent anxiety and depression care. In some countries, this is even more problematic when the authority to prescribe psychoactive medications is limited to psychiatrists.

Practices in the Middle East

Screening

Anxiety and depression are extremely common. Anxiety and depression can also be treated, to great benefit for the adolescent patient. Thus, every adolescent should be screened for anxiety and depression at least annually. For anxiety, the GAD-7 is a proven and available screening tool available in English (https://adaa.org/sites/default/files/GAD-7_Anxiety-updated_0.pdf) and in other languages (https://www.phqscreeners.com/select-screener). For depression, the PHQ-9 is similarly available in English (https://med.stanford.edu/fastlab/research/imapp/msrs/_jcr_content/main/accordion/accordion_content3/download_256324296/file.res/PHQ9%20id%20date%2008.03.pdf) and other languages (https://www.phqscreeners.com/select-screener). Screening should be considered more frequently for adolescents with symptoms suggestive of a mental health disorder and can also be used to follow the course of symptoms over time.

Screening with positive results should be followed by one-on-one clinical assessment to accurately make relevant clinical diagnoses. The websites listed for the English versions also provide numerical guidance to determine the severity of the condition.

Managing and Referring Adolescents with Anxiety and/or Depression

Most management of adolescent anxiety and depression will be done by pediatricians and primary care clinicians. Only those individuals with moderate-to severe or refractory symptoms should require input from a psychiatrist. However, institution of psychological therapies and medications is complicated, and referral is appropriate whenever the primary clinician does not have adequate experience to provide such care.

Once a clinical diagnosis is confirmed and comorbid medical conditions (such as thyroid disease, iron deficiency, and anemia) are treated, care can be initiated. Of course, comorbid mental health conditions such as attention deficit disorder and autism spectrum disorder should also be managed.

Mild anxiety and depression can sometimes be managed with active support and, usually, cognitive behavioral therapy. More aggressive intervention is reserved for those with more significant symptoms.

Therapy

Feelings, thoughts, and behaviors are all intertwined. Negative thoughts (sometimes referred to as cognitive distortions) prompt bad feelings and self-destructive behaviors. Cognitive behavioral therapy (CBT) focuses on modifying negative thinking and reducing unhelpful behaviors to alter the ongoing cycles of depression and anxiety. Cognitive behavior therapy is helpful in decreasing symptoms and improving function in adolescents with all degrees of anxiety and depression and should be offered to every affected adolescent.

With cognitive behavioral therapy, the adolescent is guided to learn to reduce and restructure negative thoughts and thought processes and to activate good behaviors by positive attention to self-care, regular sleep and meal schedules, and appropriate exercise. Diaphragmatic breathing and relaxation strategies can also support cognitive behavioral therapy. Professional guidance in cognitive behavioral therapy can continue through repeated sessions (perhaps ten to 20 sessions) over time. While cognitive behavioral therapy is usually provided by a trained psychologist, other clinicians can develop expertise with the techniques, and some online resources can be helpful.

Cognitive behavioral therapy is sometimes summarized as a three-step process: (1) identify negative and unhelpful thoughts and thought processes, (2) intentionally replace unhelpful thoughts with true, positive thoughts, and, (3) allow repeated helpful thoughts to become habitual in what some call a "re-fire to re-wire" process of strengthening healthy brain networks. For instance, when a teen is confronted by a minor challenge during daily situations and has previously responded with "see, it never works out for me" or "I just can't do anything right" can plan and implement new responses such as "I've seen this sort of situation before and know to stay calm and try a different approach."

Mental health disorders and relationships are also intertwined. Interpersonal therapy (IPT) focuses on altering dysfunctional relationships and, thus, decreasing symptoms and impairment related to depression and anxiety. Interpersonal therapy sometimes involves family members as the adolescent learns to better solve problems, process emotions, manage stress, and engage socially.

Sometimes, anxiety and depression were triggered by life experiences, and sometimes adolescents struggle to adapt to a "new normal" as their identity, importance, and independence are challenged by life situations. In these situations, acceptance and commitment therapy (ACT) can be useful. The adolescent is encouraged to *accept* situations that are beyond personal control and then to *commit* to taking positive steps to make favorable behavioral changes to improve daily functioning.

For adolescents with specific anxiety-triggering situations or objects, exposure desensitization therapy can help. With professional guidance, the adolescent learns to tolerate gradually increasing contact with the anxiety-triggering agent or activity.

All types of therapy should be accompanied by improvements in daily habits. Appropriate meals and dietary intake, regular adequate sleep, daily physical exercise, and frequent unstructured social activities should be encouraged.

> **An Illustrative Case from My Practice**
> A 15-year-old girl showed increased withdrawal over 2–3 years, isolating herself in her room and avoiding family interactions. Despite longer sleeping hours, she wakes up tired, has lost interest in her previous hobbies and her friends, and has a constant low mood and decreased appetite. The girl exhibits symptoms and signs of depression, suicidal thoughts and self-harm that was identified by clinical history, screening tools, and physical examination. She was sent to see a psychologist for cognitive behavioral therapy and was started on escitalopram 5 mg daily with planned follow-up.
>
> Madeeha Kamal, MBCHB, FAAP, FRCP
> Doha, Qatar

Medications

When anxiety and depression are moderately or severely symptomatic with functional impairment, treatment with medication should be considered. Several medications are available in most countries and are widely recommended. Some significantly impaired adolescents need to have the helpful effect of medication before cognitive behavioral therapy is fully effective.

For depression, a first-choice medication would be a selective serotonin reuptake inhibitor (SSRI) such as fluoxetine (usually starting at 10 mg once daily and, if needed, increasing over two to six weeks to 20 or even 40 mg) or escitalopram (starting at 5 mg and increasing over two to six weeks to 10 or even 20 mg as needed). Sertraline would be another option, pending availability and approval in the specific country of use. If there has not been adequate improvement by six weeks after the last dosage increase, the medication could be weaned, and an alternative SSRI antidepressant initiated. (Paroxetine is not recommended for adolescents due to greater risks of adverse reactions.) If none of the SSRIs is adequately helpful, a switch to a different medication, such as a serotonin norepinephrine reuptake inhibitor (SNRI, such as venlafaxine) or an atypical antidepressant (such as bupropion), could be considered, perhaps with input from a psychiatrist.

For anxiety, SSRIs fluoxetine and escitalopram (doses as for depression, above) and then perhaps SNRI venlafaxine) are good options. Sertraline is effective for anxiety but might prompt increased suicidal ideation in adolescents with concurrent depression.

There have been a few rare instances of increased suicidal ideation with the initiation of SSRI treatment, but the beneficial effects usually far outweigh the risk of adverse reactions. For all adolescents with depression, whether on an SSRI or not, careful follow-up is warranted—in conjunction with good observation at home, non-availability of weapons or pills potentially used for self-harm, and a "contract" by which the clinician and patient agree that, in the event of significant suicidal thinking, the patient will seek immediate help prior to initiating any self-harm.

An Illustrative Case from My Practice

A 16-year-old boy, diagnosed with autism spectrum disorder since early childhood has been struggling both academically and socially. His father, makes him feel humiliated. The boy came to my clinic in tears, asking for assistance in making friends and requesting intervention to stop his father's public insults. The family was seen by the social worker and psychologist to address parenting skills and improve communication skills, the boy was started on escitalopram, and a follow-up visit showed improvement in his mood as well as the father-child relationship.

Madeeha Kamal, MBCHB, FAAP, FRCP
Doha, Qatar

Advocacy

Realizing that adolescent anxiety and depression are becoming markedly more common in resourced societies, clinicians can also advocate for community-wide changes. Through individual, community, or even governmental involvement, clinicians involved with adolescents can advocate for societal shifts toward more unstructured play for children and less social media engagement for adolescents. Access to social media is not necessary prior to age 13 years, and continuous interruptions by social media notifications should be blocked. Simply requiring smart phones to be locked up during school hours and during the final 30 minutes before bedtime can lead to marked reductions in mental health symptoms and to significant improvements in academic and social functioning.

Note Doses of medications are mentioned in this chapter and elsewhere in this book as a general guide. While the statements in this chapter are current at the time of publication, updated resources for dosing of specific patients should be consulted prior to initiating therapy. All treatment of individual patients should be customized to the patient's particular situation.

For Reflection

What processes would be required to make regular screening for anxiety and depression possible in your clinic setting? How could you implement those processes?

Further Reading

1. Shorey S, Ng ED, Wong CHJ. Global prevalence of depression and elevated depressive symptoms among adolescents: a systematic review and meta-analysis. Br J Clin Psychol. 2022;61(2):287–305. https://doi.org/10.1111/bjc.12333.
2. Tang MH, Pinsky EG. Mood and affect disorders. Pediatr Rev. 2015;36(2):52–60.
3. Zuckerbrot RA, Cheung A, Jensen PS, REK S, Laraque D, GLAD-PC Steering Group. Guidelines for adolescent depression in primary care (GLAD-PC): part I. Practice preparation, identification, assessment, and initial management. Pediatrics. 2018;141(3):e20174081. https://publications.aap.org/pediatrics/article/141/3/e20174081/37626/Guidelines-for-Adolescent-Depression-in-Primary
4. Cheung AH, Zuckerbrot RA, Jensen PS, Laraque D, REK S, GLAD-PC Steering Group. Guidelines for adolescent depression in primary care (GLAD-PC): part II. Treatment and ongoing management. Pediatrics. 2018;141(3):e20174082. https://publications.aap.org/pediatrics/article/141/3/e20174082/37654/Guidelines-for-Adolescent-Depression-in-Primary
5. Doyle MM. Anxiety disorders in children. Pediatr Rev. 2022;43(11):618–30.
6. Haidt J. The anxious generation. Penguin Press; 2024.

Chapter 8
Concluding Comments

Thanks for joining us on the journey that is *Adolescent Medicine in the Middle East*. It's been a pleasure to share life with you as we wrote these pages and, now, as you read these pages. The journey continues as, together, we seek to implement the principles, perspectives, and practices discussed in this book for the good of adolescents in the Middle East.

In fact, the physical presence of this book is the result of a five-year gestation. We could rightly claim that the book was conceived shortly after one of us (PRF) arrived in the United Arab Emirates in 2020. Then, there was only one person trained in adolescent medicine practicing in the country, and adolescents often felt excluded from medical care systems. Hospitals and clinics were still deciding which doctors should care for teenagers, and many pediatricians lacked experience dealing with patients older than 15 years of age. It didn't take long to realize that the UAE was actually ahead of some other countries in the region since it already had one adolescent medicine consultant and since the country was grappling with how best to train pediatric residents to care for older adolescents.

On the other hand, we could rightly claim that this book began when two of the three of us authors were personally growing into the adolescent years in the Middle East. Combined, over recent decades, the three of us have spent time in nearly every Middle Eastern country, and we value collaboration with colleagues throughout the region.

This book is, in fact, the result of our combined 150 years of experience in the Middle East and throughout the world; it is also the result of our passionate desire to see adolescents thriving throughout the Middle East. This book is a gift to the current and coming generations of clinicians who will care for adolescents in the Middle East. What we have lived and learned has been shared in this book so others can extend our experience to even better care for future patients.

During the five-year-long "gestation" of this book, the world has changed, too. The COVID-19 pandemic worsened and then faded into history. Artificial (or augmented) intelligence (AI) has moved from the frontier of future possibilities to daily

A. J. Chattha et al., *Adolescent Medicine in the Middle East: Principles,
Perspectives, Practices*, https://doi.org/10.1007/978-3-032-12348-0_8

practice. Information is readily available in overwhelming detail. Thus, we have tried to avoid overwhelming readers with yet more detail; rather, our goal was to go beyond facts, to discuss the principles and perspectives that can guide daily evidence-based practice. We hope that is useful to each of you who is reading and using this book.

We also realize that adolescent medicine is not a solo endeavor; it is a "team sport." The three of us joined together to produce the book, harnessing our varied backgrounds and experiences in different parts of the Middle East. And we did this as friends and colleagues, having worked together at the Mayo Clinic even before that institution established itself in the Arabian Peninsula. As you have seen in these pages, we also engaged other colleagues who provided peer review of early drafts of the chapters in this book and who added their own helpful comments to the text.

Now, the teamwork continues. You get to take and use the material in this book as you incorporate our ideas in ways that fit with your practice. Together, we aim to better serve the adolescents of the future. Thanks for journeying with us, and thanks for extending the journey into clinics and hospitals and countries throughout the Middle East.

Index

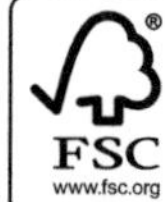

FSC
www.fsc.org
MIX
Papier aus verantwortungsvollen Quellen
Paper from responsible sources
FSC® C105338